T0373652

In-patient Mental Health Care from the Asylum System to the Present Day

With a focus on the progression and dismantlement of the asylum system, this book examines key issues around the policy and practice of in-patient mental health provision in the UK, making comparisons with similar services in other parts of the world.

Part narrative history and critical analysis, part autoethnography, this unique volume critiques the ethics of early policy decisions which led to the closure of the old Victorian asylums and the advent of care in the community, identifying continuing issues of institutionalisation, containment and segregation. Drawing parallels with the continuing dilemmas of 'inclusion' in other areas of public policy and provision, chapters discuss controversial issues such as the response to the Covid-19 pandemic, the influence of 'anti-psychiatry' and the continuing use of electroconvulsive therapy. Ultimately, the book makes a vital theoretical and practical contribution to the continuing debate around in-patient mental health care in the 21st century.

The book will be of interest to academics, researchers and policymakers in the fields of healthcare policy and history of mental health provision more broadly. Psychiatrists interested in the history of the asylum system in the UK, as well as present-day mental health professionals, will also find the book of use.

Andrew Colley is former Senior Lecturer at the University of East London, UK. This is his third book published by Routledge after *Inclusion is Dead, Long Live Inclusion* (2017), co-authored with Peter Imray, and *Enhancing Wellbeing and Independence for Young People with Profound and Multiple Learning Difficulties* (2022), co-authored with Julie Tilbury.

Advances in Mental Health Research
Books in this series:

In-patient Mental Health Care from the Asylum System to the Present Day

A Lived Experience of Policy and Practice

Andrew Colley

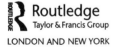

LONDON AND NEW YORK

First published 2024
by Routledge
4 Park Square, Milton Park, Abingdon, Oxon OX14 4RN

and by Routledge
605 Third Avenue, New York, NY 10158

Routledge is an imprint of the Taylor & Francis Group, an informa business

British Library Cataloguing-in-Publication Data
A catalogue record for this book is available from the British Library

ISBN: 978-1-032-59289-3 (hbk)
ISBN: 978-1-032-59511-5 (pbk)
ISBN: 978-1-003-45504-2 (ebk)

DOI: 10.4324/9781003455042

Typeset in Times New Roman
by Apex CoVantage, LLC

Contents

Acknowledgements

I am grateful to the following people for their invaluable help with the research and writing of this book:

Maggie Batchelar
Michelle Burke
Rebecca Blackstone
Caroline Clarke
Allison Darken
Tracey Holland
Dr Janet Hoskin
Sarah Kingston
John Neil
Penny Newman
Dr Katy Pepper
Nicholas Ruber
Anna Russell
Sarah Weeks
Amy Wright

And to Gillian and Sam, who put up with me through thick and thin, sanity and madness. Thank you and sorry.

Prologue

Into the cage

It is a few weeks before Christmas 2020. My belongings are bundled into bin liners by four people I don't know who came into my room unannounced in the night. Later, weeks later, I will notice what has gone missing. Nothing particularly sentimental, certainly nothing valuable: just clothes really, like those pyjamas my wife brought me last month.

I may have been told earlier what was going to happen, but it made no impression on me. My wife told me later that I had rung her in tears to tell her I was being taken somewhere else, somewhere much further from my home, but I don't remember that conversation.

I am led along the long corridor by these people I don't know, as if they are bodyguards. Like a celebrity, or a criminal, or what I actually am. Some of the other 'service users,' as we are told we are, are standing at their doors or outside the nursing station. *Where's he going?*, one asks. *He's fucked*, says another. A nurse joins the front of our little procession to open the three sets of security doors which lead to the loading bay where a minibus is waiting. The back doors are opened, and I am invited to step inside.

Except this isn't an ordinary minibus, because as I climb in through the back doors, I realise I will not be sitting in one of the seats with the others. The end of the minibus, a section no more than 2 feet long and barely the width of the minibus itself, has been turned into a cage. A lattice of bars separates me from the rest of the seating area. In fact, there are bars all around me. There is no seat, just a low metal bench screwed to the floor with no back rest. Only the bars to lean against, and no seat belt.

A heavy metal sliding door is closed and locked and the minibus doors closed and locked behind that. No one joins me in this cage. I look through the bars into the body of the minibus. The bin liners containing my things are thrown through the side doors, and the four people who have brought me here climb in. With the driver, that makes five people – five people just for me: a 62-year-old professional man. With a wife, a son and a house with a garden in the countryside not far away from here. Five people. What for? To protect me? I don't think so. To stop me escaping? Unlikely from this cage. To protect each other from me? Possibly, but why? I have never harmed anyone in my life. And as the bus lurches off into the night, I feel, even through the fog of illness and medication, and not for the first or the last time in those dreadful months, humiliated.

The radio is turned on. Music. The five people in the minibus chat, laugh, doze and watch me. They haven't spoken to me since they first came into my room, the room which had held me for the last ten weeks, a room which was even now being stripped, cleaned and disinfected for the next person. There are no windows out of my cage, and I can only look up through the internal bars, into the minibus and watch streetlights flash by outside the side windows. I think I know this road. I have driven it many times, for work, to visit friends and relatives, but this time I am on a darker journey and one I have not chosen. I guess now where we are going: from one county town in England to another. It's about 25 miles but the minibus is slow. It is an uncomfortable journey, for so many reasons, but for that hour mainly physically as I try to balance on my small metal bench with my back being jolted against the bars of my cage.

The bus begins to make some turns, lights outside become brighter and more frequent. The other people in the bus begin to stir. A couple wake up. We have arrived. The back doors open. We are parked outside a reception area which looks very similar to the one we left about an hour ago.

Two people are waiting. They are wearing those 'not uniforms' people in the NHS and other care settings often wear these days. Dark blue, plain. Not a uniform but not something you'd wear on a night out. The only signpost to their jobs are the bright NHS lanyards round their necks. They are 'double masked,' that is to say a visor over a blue face mask, but I've got used to this.

It must be the early hours of the morning. I don't have a watch – anymore. The people in the not uniforms seem anxious to take me inside, but before they do, I am approached by the driver of the minibus. He is carrying a clipboard and a pen which he hands to me.

Before you go, could you just fill in this short customer satisfaction form please?

Of course I will. It's what I am like, or used to be: compliant, happy to help. Nice. He was right: it's not a long form at all. One page of A4 with boxes and big writing. One of those ordinal scale questionnaires which ask you to rate your satisfaction on a scale from 1 to 4: *How was the service you received today? To what extent did you feel your needs were met?* I fill it in under the light outside the reception area, average scores: 2: quite satisfied, 3: satisfied. I think most people do that with these types of questionnaires. The easiest answers. Don't want to rock the boat, though I don't remember seeing some

of the most common questions on these forms. Questions like: *Would you recommend this service to others? How likely are you to use this service again?*
I do remember the last question though:

How do you think we could improve the service provided to you today?

I didn't answer that one. I sensed the care staff were getting impatient. They wanted me up on the ward and in bed. In a way though, this book is my attempt to answer that question. It's not about my own mental health, except when I can't avoid it to discuss policy and practice as I experienced them, and it certainly isn't a self-help or well-being book. It won't try to tell anyone how to avoid getting ill or how to get well. It's a book about how in-patient care got to where it is today, and why: the good things and the bad, and it's about how we might 'improve the service provided.' And it's also about how in-patient mental health wards coped with the biggest crisis in the NHS's 80-year history: the Covid pandemic.

1 Psychiatric hospitals in the 19th and 20th centuries

This book is about adult in-patient mental health care. By 'in-patient care' in this context it is meant the care of those whose mental health has deteriorated to such an extent that it is in their best interests to stay for a while in a hospital, although as we will see, the words used to describe this type of residential provision, and those who use it, change over time.

The book focuses on a period of about 40 years from the 1980s to the present day and discusses how the policy and practice of in-patient care have evolved in that time in England, drawing comparisons with other countries of the world, and in particular the United States. The book is based, to a large extent, on first-hand accounts. The voices of a number of service users and some staff will be heard, but the primary lived experience will be that of the author, who received in-patient care in hospitals in England in 1985 and again in 2020. This 35-year gap meant that the author experienced both the asylum system which was still in place in the 1980s and in-patient mental health care as it exists today: in smaller units often attached to general hospitals. The social, cultural and economic background to changes in provision over time are discussed, and accounts of lived experience are compared with academic research and placed in the context of policy and legislation. The final chapters ask what have we gained and what have we lost since the end of the asylum system, discuss barriers to change and look to the future with proposals for better in-patient care.

The terminology used in the book reflects the language in use at different times and as Filer (2019) reminds us 'there is no uncontroversial language when talking about mental illness – and that includes the phrase *mental illness*' (p. 5), though happily we have moved on from phrases such as *Colony for the Mentally Defective*, which is engraved on the remains of an old stone gatepost in the grounds of what was Aycliffe Hospital in County Durham in the UK. Some of the historic language of in-patient care is difficult to read and hear, and inverted commas are used in the first instance to show where terms have been taken from historical records and other sources.

This first chapter sets the scene by briefly charting the history and practice of in-patient mental health care from the beginning of formalised provision

DOI: 10.4324/9781003455042-1

in the 17th century to the end of the 20th century when some of the significant changes took place which have impacted on in-patient care today. The author's lived experience is expressed in the first person.

My first encounter with what are often called the 'Victorian asylums' was not as a patient in the 1980s but as a delivery driver for a firm of printers on the outskirts of London nearly a decade earlier. One of my tasks was to deliver occupational therapy work for in-patients in some of the large psychiatric hospitals which Clair Wills, writing in *The London Review of Books* in November 2021, described as being 'hung like beads around the neck of Outer London' (p. 23). They were not called 'asylums' by then, but 'asylum' was still a term in common usage, alongside other more demeaning phrases. The names of these hospitals – Friern, Netherne, Cane Hill and many others – are now lost or, as we will see later in the book, reappropriated and re-purposed. They were imposing places covering acres of land with usually one main building and different wards linked by one long corridor. Often there was a chapel, and a water tower, which as we will discuss, became a potent symbol in debates over future provision, but at the time was simply built because the 'ready availability of a large volume of water was vital for tackling a fire' (McCrae, 2016, p. 16). There were also often other 'units' – often called 'houses,' even 'villas' – in the grounds: for the young, the very old or for those who were 'difficult to manage' which could include those we now describe as having autistic spectrum condition (ASC) or learning difficulties. Despite the separation of learning difficulty from mental illness in the landscape of social care in the last 40 years, we will see in Chapter 7 that the placement of people with special needs in psychiatric wards has resurfaced today.

In one of these hospitals, Earlswood near Redhill in Surrey, I met Nerissa and Katherine Bowes-Lyon, the first cousins of the late Queen Elizabeth II. I handed one of them a pile of envelopes to fill with advertising material. She thanked me graciously. Most people involved with Earlswood Hospital at the time knew Nerissa and Katherine were there, but it would be years before tabloid newspapers and a Channel 4 documentary revealed their existence. More recently, in Series 4, Episode 7 of the Netflix Docudrama *The Crown* (2020), their bleak lives in the hospital were contrasted with the lavish lifestyles of their close family. It is an accurate depiction of the hospital as I witnessed it: a smoke-filled room with high windows, patients slumped in chairs, laughing, crying; games of cards, pots of tea, birthday cakes, though when I talked for the purposes of this book to the brother of a woman who was on the same ward as the Bowes-Lyon sisters, he said that his own abiding memories are of the stone staircases, communal toilets and long drafty, noisy corridors.

I also took work to Cane Hill Hospital near Croydon, now a London Borough. There was a ward there full of men in their 60s and 70s speaking in a language I didn't understand. I asked one of the nurses who they were. She explained that they were all Polish airmen who had enlisted in the RAF in the Second World War. They had been traumatised in one way or another by their wartime experiences, had lost contact or been rejected by their families back in Poland and had never returned. They seemed happy in this home away from home: chatting, singing, playing board games. Cane Hill Hospital was their home, and they were cared for and loved by the staff there.

Without realising it at the time, I was witnessing both the good and the bad of the 'asylum system' as it had existed for more than 200 years in the UK: on the one hand, a convenient place to hide away the relatives you no longer want to look after or are embarrassed to acknowledge, and on the other hand, a place of safety for sick and vulnerable people with nowhere else to go. As we will see throughout this book, these dichotomies and many others like them still exist within mental health provision in the 21st century. The Queen's cousins are long dead, but the fractured nature of family and social ties in Britain today mean that for some, in-patient mental health care still acts as an 'asylum' away from a community or a family that has served them poorly and in which they can't for the moment cope. We will discuss these issues in greater depth later in this book.

So, what were these 'asylums'? Where had they come from and why? What purpose had they served? There have been many books tracing the history of the asylums in the UK and abroad and of these, Barbara Taylor's extraordinary *The Last Asylum* (2014) and Sarah Wise's *Inconvenient People* (2013) provide concise accounts of provision in the UK. Andrew Scull's *Madness in Civilisation* (2015) and Mike Jay's *This Way Madness Lies* (2016) place these institutions in the context of our understanding of mental illness as a whole, and Kathleen Jones' rigorously researched *Asylums and After: A Revised History of the Mental Health Services: From the Early 18th Century to the 1990s* (1993) looks in depth at much of the complex policy background to current provision. I am indebted to all these books and many other sources. For the purposes of this chapter however, we only need to provide a brief timeline up to last decades of the 20th century when the concept of asylums for the mentally unwell, and the asylums themselves, began to crumble.

For many centuries, 'most lunatics lived with their families or roamed the countryside' (Taylor, 2014, p. 105) but in 1676, Bethlem Hospital – commonly referred to as 'Bedlam' – became 'England's first purpose-built hospital for the insane' (ibid., p. 105), and was only closed to sightseers and tourists over a century later. The 18th century saw 'the nascent shift towards an embrace of the asylum as the preferred solution to the problems the lunatic posed' (Scull, 2015, p. 189) and the growth in charity or more usually privately funded 'madhouses.' These became a 'lucrative business for owners' (ibid., p. 105) as well as in some cases places of abuse and neglect.

The Government really acted only twice in the 18th century to address issues around mental health, and this relatively low frequency of Government action compared to other public sectors such as education is something we will see continuing into the 21st century. The Vagrancy Acts of 1714 and 1744 made a distinction between 'lunatics' and 'other undesirables,' and also protected lunatics from public whippings, though vagrants it seems were still fair game. In 1774, the 'Act for the regulation of private madhouses' brought in compulsory licensing of all madhouses accommodating more than one lunatic and 'Lunacy Commissioners' granted these licences. But despite these minor Government interventions, at the beginning of the 19th century, in-patient care was still big business with Brislington House Asylum outside Bristol, which segregated patients not only by gender but also by social class, charging as much as £300 per annum, which equates to over £30K today (Wise, 2013), though it too was not immune to allegations of abuse.

The beginning of the large publicly funded asylums can be traced back to 1807 and a House of Commons inquiry into the state of lunacy in England that recommended establishment of county asylums funded by the 'poor rates,' which was a tax levied on property to fund the relief of poverty and other social causes. The Lunacy Act (Inspection of Asylums) and the County Asylums Act of 1845 led to the requirement for every county in England to build an asylum, though Scotland resisted this and tried to keep their lunatics in families, but were eventually overruled by Westminster (Scull, 2015). The ethos and design of many of the asylums of this time – both publicly and privately funded – were influenced by the idea of 'moral treatment' pioneered by the Quakers at the York Retreat which had opened in 1796. The pioneers of this kinder approach to mental health care argued that an asylum should be a symbol of civilisation but without the stressful bits: providing a humane and caring environment where those that could not cope with the world outside would find respite (Scull, p. 205). An asylum would be 'exactly what the word originally meant – a place of refuge from a very harsh world' (Jones, 1993, p. 40). It was also around this time that we find the first manifestation of organised advocacy for service users with the founding of the 'Alleged Lunatics' Friend Society.'

The 1845 Lunatics Act required that all patients confined in licensed institutions had to be certified as insane before their confinement (Shepherd & Wright, 2002) so that it became less possible for families to engineer the confinement of 'difficult' relatives with no medical justification simply by petitioning local magistrates. Physical restraint and confinement though remained common, and 'by the late 1860's most asylums had reintroduced straitjacketing and other physical restraints' (Taylor, 2014, p. 110). The balance between care and confinement, restraint and recovery will be a theme of in-patient mental health care to this day, and of this book, though cruelty as in this account from the casebooks of Brooklands Asylum from 1871, cited in Shepherd and Wright (2002), is now much rarer:

> She was brought in a canvas garment which fitted her person even down to her ankles, the arms however not going through the sleeves, but being folded across her chest close to her skin, the hands being locked in leather gloves. The jacket being [fastened] at the back by 5 locks.
>
> (Casebooks (Female) Brookwood Asylum, 1871)

These hospital records are often the nearest we can get to the lived experience of patients at the time, though Berkencotter (2011) uncovered the testimony of one Walter Marshall who was detained in the Ticehurst Asylum in East Sussex in 1876 and who witnessed 'an old man treated very cruelly' (Minutes of Evidence, p. 420).

The second half of the 19th century also saw the birth in Britain of psychiatry as a profession, the word 'psychiatrist' gradually replacing the French term 'alienists' who were also often the owners of the institutions themselves. This professionalisation, but also medicalisation, of treatment was reinforced by the Lunacy Act of 1890 which defined even more clearly the terms for the certification of asylums and the detention of patients. It 'appeared primarily to protect society' (McCrae, 2016, p. 44), whereas previous lunacy laws 'arose from concern at the plight of the mentally disordered' (ibid.). The Act remained in force for an extraordinary 69 years until it was repealed by the Mental Health Act 1959, at which point the term 'moral defective' was finally replaced.

The end of the 19th century and the very early years of the 20th century were the highpoint for the building of these asylums. Friern, known then as Colney Hatch, was opened in 1850, Earlswood in 1855, Banstead in 1877, Cane Hill in 1882 and Netherne Hospital, which we will visit in Chapter 3, in 1905. These large institutions were built on land which was 'fruitful, with sufficient acreage and livestock for ample crops, meat and dairy produce' (McCrae, 2016, p. 9). They had their own farms, police force, fire brigade, electric generators and graveyards (Scull, 2015). Some also had their own railway line.

During and after the First World War, the asylums accommodated tens of thousands of traumatised soldiers. With many of them still on the wards years later, the Mental Treatment Act of 1930 arguably softened the language and framing of mental illness by removing the word 'lunatic' and replacing the word 'asylum' with 'hospital.' The categories of 'voluntary' and 'temporary' patients were also introduced prefiguring categories used today.

As the Second World War was dragging to a conclusion, with more men and women returning home scarred by their experiences, initial plans for the National Health Service (NHS) in England and the devolved countries of Scotland, Wales and Northern Ireland were set out, but excluded mental health services, though mental hospitals were incorporated into the NHS at its foundation in 1948. By 1947, the National Council for Civil Liberties – which had been funded in 1934 – estimated that there were 54,000 people 'confined' in hospitals, a figure close to the 53,337 new detentions under the Mental Health Act recorded in 2021–2022 (NHS, 2022).

Services for the mentally ill developed at different speeds and in different ways in other countries over a similar period, though for some areas of the world it is difficult to find research into the history of in-patient care, and what evidence there is suggests that the responsibility for the care of the insane fell on the family, or on no one at all. The role of the state in funding asylums, and the 'great confinement of the insane that remained so notably a feature of the Western response to mental disorder until the last decades of the 20th century' (Scull p. 190) would not touch some parts of the world till much later.

By the middle of the 19th century, Europe had become a patchwork 'in which every phase of the asylum's history co-existed' (Jay, p. 106). France launched a scheme in 1819 to create a national system of asylums, but by 1852 only seven had actually been built (Scull, 2015). The first new public asylum in Austria was not built until 1853, whilst the relative political fragmentation of Italy and Germany meant that they were late to the table. In 1864, Carlo Livi, an eminent alienist, complained that asylum provision in Italy was the most backward in Europe (Scull, 2015), with Venice hosting what was known as an 'island of the mad' on San Servolo: a dreary and almost windowless place (Scull, 2015). Germany fared better, and at Alt-Scherbitz asylum (McCrae, 2016), there were gardens instead of exercise yards and lanes instead of corridors. In the Belgian town of Geel, the church of St Dymphna had for centuries taken in wandering lunatics and entrusted their care to local families. By the 19th century, the town itself had become a kind of 'community asylum' in which moral treatment was 'patched into society at large . . . with the mad wandering freely around the town' (Jay, 2016, p. 107). The town's pioneering approach to a more humane treatment of the mentally ill persists to this day. However, stigma around mental illness, particularly amongst the more well-off, meant that across Europe 'the bourgeois flight from the asylum' (Jay, 2016, p. 12) led to a new golden age for the spa, especially in the French Pyrenees and the Swiss and German Alps, and asylums, often rebranded as 'sanatoria,' advertised openly in London and Paris.

In the former colonies of many European countries, an asylum system of sorts eventually grew in the image of the movement in England, though often only for the families of the empire builders themselves and even then, the British East India Company preferred shipping its sick employees back to London (Scull, 2015) with some limited provision made for 'native' employees only later. In fact, writing in 2008, Murthy and Sekar acknowledge that 'the condition of government psychiatric hospitals in India has been a source of concern for more than a century' (2008, p. 101). In 'colonies where there was just a tiny white administrative class' (Scull, 2015, p. 199), asylums arrived much later, with the first asylums in Nigeria for instance, not open till the early 20th century. Robben Island, North of Cape Town, in South Africa, and later the place of detention of Nelson Mandela, became in the second half of the 19th century an asylum for hundreds of women judged to be insane. Elsewhere the asylum model took root in China and Japan but with China's first asylum on the Western model only opened in 1898 and Japan's in the early 1920s.

In America, although Quakers from Philadelphia had visited the York Retreat in the UK in 1813 (Jay, 2016), the political power of the individual states meant that asylum provision and practices of moral treatment advanced only slowly and as late as the 1860s it was still possible in some states to have someone committed to an asylum with no medical evidence whatsoever. In the early decades of the 20th century, the American asylums remained primarily places of confinement and restraint where little had changed in the past 100 years. Emily Holmes Coleman, for instance, in a fictionalised account of her own actual confinement in an asylum in New York in 1930 describes being forcibly restrained in a full-body canvas straightjacket with just a hole for the head, very similar to the one from the casebooks of Brooklands Asylum cited earlier.

Gradually though, in both America and Europe, the asylums were also becoming theatres for experimentation. In 1936, the American neurologist Walter Freeman bored holes in the frontal lobes of a patient in an early lobotomy. In 1938, the use of electric shocks to the brain was developed by the Italian neurologist Ugo Cerletti after he witnessed the technique used on a pig in an abattoir in Rome, and at around the same time German, Austrian, French and British psychiatrists were using electric currents on their patients to 'get the mute to speak, the deaf to hear and the lame to walk' (Scull, 2015, p. 297). We will hear a modern-day lived experience of electroconvulsive therapy (ECT) at the end of this book.

As in Britain, all over Europe asylums were requisitioned to house the psychic casualties of the century's world wars, though particularly in the second conflict some also became sites of deadly purpose. Some notable German psychiatrists 'had been enthusiastic proponents of eugenics in the 1920s' (Scull, 2015, p. 258) and their skewed logic drew conclusions with respect to those with mental illnesses. In October 1939, shortly after the invasion of Poland, hundreds of inmates of a mental hospital in Owińska just North of Poznan were murdered (Barham, 2020), and in the same month Hitler launched the so-called T-4 programmes: the disabled and mentally ill were rounded up and sent to a number of hospitals, where they were exterminated (Scull, 2015). In France, the excess mortality rate in psychiatric hospitals during the occupation was staggering (von Bueltzingsloewen, 2002) and thousands of the mentally ill died of starvation during the German occupation (ibid.). Jews in psychiatric hospitals all over occupied Europe found themselves 'at the confluence of eugenics, Christian anti-Judaism, and the racist and anti-Semitic mania of the Nazis' (Mouchenik & Fau-Vincenti, 2019, p. 545) and few survived.

After these wartime horrors, to a certain extent 'the purpose of the hospitals shifted from being primarily custodial towards the goals of treatment and care' (Wills, 2021, p. 24), and in England at least 'in the early post-war years mental hospitals acquired a mixture of the ethos of the public school and a holiday camp' (Jones, 1993, p. 146), with 'entertainments, film shows, ward parties, and games of cricket or football at neighbouring asylums' (Barham, 2020, p. 1). However, this perhaps rose-tinted post-war age was short-lived. By the mid-1950s, the asylum population in the UK reached a peak (Scull,

2015) of nearly 160,000, whilst in the United States during the same period, the asylum population was nearly four times as high (ibid.). Asylums again became increasingly associated – in the public consciousness at least – with abuse, punishment and physical restraint. These issues would continue to dominate policy into the 21st century, arguably at the expense of more pragmatic debates around the care and well-being of the patients.

The early 1950s also marked the first use of psychotropic drugs, with Scull (2015) noting that 'if they were not the first cause of deinstitutionalisation, their advent did nonetheless transform psychiatry' (p. 378), though Main in an early paper 'The Ailment' (1957) discussed a study on an in-patient ward in which it was discovered that nurses tended to give sedation when they, the nursing staff, could not cope any more.

The prevailing post-war ethos, the 'period of conscious decolonization' (Wall, 2018, p. 4), alongside the development of new medications, would finally lead by the end of the century to the decommissioning of the large asylums. In the UK, the 1959 Mental Health Act finally repealed the Lunacy Act of 1890 and arguably marked the first step in the dismantling of the asylums with its stress on 'the desirability of avoiding institutional care' (Jack, 1998, p. 27), and as the 1960s dawned, the mission of psychiatry to 'quarantine the uncurable rather than restoring them to sanity' (Scull, 2015, p. 303) was being increasingly called into question. With the growth of talking therapies, shock therapies and psychosurgery were 'assailed as symbols of psychiatric oppression' (Scull, 2015, p. 318). The French philosopher Michel Foucault dismissed the idea that asylums could be in any way humane, and the Canadian American sociologist Ervin Goffman in his book *Asylums* (1961) regarded the asylum as a special case of a closed society which manipulated its members into pathological behaviours. In the UK, David Cooper, one of the prime movers of the anti-psychiatry movement which we will discuss in the next chapter, compared mental hospitals to Nazi concentration camps arguing that they serve the same function of destroying people's humanity (Wall, 2016), and Russell Barton, who was superintendent of Severalls Mental Hospital in Kent and later head of the Rochester Psychiatric Centre in New York, coined the term 'institutional neurosis' to describe the harmful effects of long-term confinement (Scull, 2015).

Powerful political voices were also being raised against the old asylums. Much has been written about a speech made in 1961 by Enoch Powell, the British Minister for Health in the Conservative Government of Harold Mac-Millan. Powell's speech is sometimes considered to have fired the starting gun for the closure of the asylums but as we have seen, the process was already gaining ground. Powell's speech though was certainly heavy with anti-asylum rhetoric, calling for the almost total 'elimination' of these hospitals, 'brooded over by the gigantic water-tower and chimney combined' and the 'redundancy' of at least 75,000 beds. These 'isolated institutions' would be 'doomed' by the 'assault' he was leading, which he acknowledged had 'almost become an obsession' for him.

However, as even Powell had acknowledged, there were and always would be people whose illness was so severe, who represented a danger to themselves or to others, or whose difficulties in coping with the community meant that they needed to spend time in hospital. Powell's suggestion was that they may have to remain in the old hospitals, and for a time that was exactly what happened, but as more and more of the buildings themselves were sold to developers, this was clearly not a long-term solution. The Hospital Plan of 1962, put forward by Powell himself, was an ambitious project to build 90 new general hospitals as well as refurbishing many more and so 'presaged the rundown of the asylums and the assimilation of psychiatric care into the wider hospital system' (Turner et al., 2015. p. 602). By the end of 1962, though, the Hospital Plan was beginning to come under scrutiny. The *Daily Herald* newspaper ran with an article by Nicholas Lloyd and John Spicer 'Calling Enoch Powell, Health Minister: Crisis in the Hospitals' and reported on a crisis of funding. By 1963, the Treasury had cut the proposed funding increase to enact the Hospital Plan from 3% to 1.5% leaving many Health Boards unable to meet the costs.

Replacement of the asylums was not 'bounding forward as Powell had envisaged' (McCrae and Nolan p. 195). It was clear that the hospitals would survive for longer than anyone had expected: for many long-stay patients, these places had been their homes and they 'did not march to the gate' (Mcrae and Nolan p. 163). They were also in some cases homes and social hubs for the nurses, many staff were resistant to change and hospital managers were in no rush to empty their wards.

The time was also ripe, in the UK at least, to repeal the 1959 Mental Health Act. The major impetus for the reform of the 1959 Act was driven by Lord 'Rab' Butler (1902–1982), the Conservative politician who was the president of the mental health charity MIND and the chairman of the Butler Committee on 'mentally abnormal offenders' which had been set up in 1972 and made its final report in 1975. These were years marked by public alarm over the release from high-security psychiatric hospitals of offenders who went on to commit further terrible crimes, and two in particular: Graham Young, released from Broadmoor in 1971 and who within a year had poisoned two work colleagues, and Terence Iliffe, who killed his wife in December 1973 after being released from detention in January of the same year.

The new Act, in the words of the secretary of state for social services, Norman Fowler, did not 'seek in any way to overturn the principles of the 1959 Act' (Fowler, 1982) but would only concern a 'small number of people whose behaviour could constitute a danger to themselves or others' (ibid.). The new Act did strengthen the protection of the civil rights of mentally ill people (Turner et al., 2015), but from its very inception it was not so much about care, as about compulsory detention and treatment, and is clearly concerned for the safety of the mentally ill and of those around them with the word 'safety,' usually within the phrase 'place of safety,' occurring nearly three times as much in 1983 than in 1959.

The word 'well-being' though occurs only once in the 1983 Act, and the word 'recovery' not at all, which is one less reference than in 1959, and it is not till Part Ten on page 100 of the new Act that 'informal admissions' (p. 92) or what were then called 'voluntary patients' are mentioned. Jones (1993) points out that the 'great majority of people with psychiatric problems, whether in hospital or out, received little or no attention from would-be reformers' (Jones, 1993. p. 215) and regrets that the 'whole debate which occupied the mental health movement for the best part of a decade was a diversion from the major task of providing effective community care for all patients' (p. 213). There would remain for the next 40 years a 'nagging sense that such a policy was not good enough for a civilised society' (Jones, 1993, p. 254), but these concerns 'could always be appeased by turning moral outrage on the old asylums' (ibid.).

Another key driver for the tone and content of the 1983 Act was the fact that it was developed and passed through Parliament at the start of the premiership of Margaret Thatcher. The Thatcherite agenda was focused on cutting public expenditure, the privatisation of NHS support services and the selling off of Government assets, and arguably the 1983 Act itself was at least in part a product of what became known as 'Thatcherism': public service provision would henceforth be 'consumer-led' (Barham, 2020, p. 145). Customer choice became 'a must-have of 20th century welfare policy' (Taylor, 2014, p. 253) and with more than 70 references to 'management' and 'administration,' arguably it is the 'business' of mental health care which, alongside safety and risk management, is at the heart of the legal framework which governs mental health care in England today.

In common with many UK Acts of Parliament, the Mental Health Act 1983 had an associated Code of Practice which can be revised by officials or by statutory Instrument. The Secretary of State for Health described this Code as being

> (a) for the guidance of registered medical practitioners, managers and staff of hospitals and mental nursing homes and approved social workers in relation to the admission of patients to hospitals and mental nursing homes under this Act; and (b) for the guidance of registered medical practitioners and members of other professions in relation to the medical treatment of patients suffering from mental disorder.
>
> (Section 118, p. 92)

So, it is to this regularly updated Code of Practice that practitioners have to turn to find guidance on the actual care and treatment of the mentally ill, irrespective of their status as compulsorily detained or informal patients. The Code of Practice is gentler in tone and content than the Act itself in its attitudes to care and is far less focused on the details of compulsory detention with 21 references to 'informal patients.' Within the Code there are also

54 references to 'dignity,' 24 to 'recovery' and it has dedicated sections on human rights, equality, privacy and aftercare. It also specifies the following five 'guiding principles' that should be considered when making all decisions in relation to care, support or treatment:

- Least restrictive option and maximising independence
- Empowerment and involvement
- Respect and dignity
- Purpose and effectiveness
- Efficiency and equity

By 1985, things were slowly changing, but much of the old world of the asylums was still in place. Before I entered one of those asylums as a patient in the dying years of that system, I would spend a short time in a sort of in-between place. A place which, though it was actively embracing the deconstruction of the asylums, was at the same time grappling with some of the ideas about mental health and treatment which flourished in the 1960s. It was a place where the old and the new collided.

References

Barham, P. (2020). *Closing the Asylum – The Mental Patient in Modern Society*. London: Process Press.

Berkencotter, C. (2011). A Patient's Tale of Incarceration in a Victorian Lunatic Asylum. *International Journal of English Studies*, 11(1), 1–14.

Coleman, E.H. (1930). *The Shutter of Snow*. New York: George Routledge and Sons Ltd.

Department of Health. (2015). *Mental Health Act 1983 Code of Practice*. London: The Stationery Office.

Filer, N. (2019). *This Book Will Change Your Mind about Mental Health*. London: Faber and Faber.

Fowler, N. (1982). *Hansard* (Volume 20). March 22nd 1982.

Jack, R. (1998). Institutions in Community Care. In Jack, R. (Ed.), *Residential Versus Community Care – The Role of Institutions in Welfare Provision*. London: MacMillan Press.

Jay, M. (2016). *This Way Madness Lies*. London: Thames and Hudson.

Jones, K. (1993). *Asylums and After: A Revised History of the Mental Health Services: From the Early 18th Century to the 1990's*. London: Athlone.

Lloyd, N., & Spicer, J. (1962). Crisis in the Hospital. *Daily Herald*. October 9th 1962.

Main, T. (1957). The Ailment. *British Journal of Medical Psychology*, 30, 129–145.

McCrae, N., & Nolan, P. (2016). *The Story of Nursing in British Mental Hospitals: Echoes from the Corridors*. Abingdon: Routledge.

Morgan, P., Wilson, J., McGonigle, M. (Writers), & Hobbs, J. (Director). In Morgan, P., Daldry, S., Harries, A., Martin, P., Mackie, S., Byam Shaw, M., Fox, R., Seghatchian, T., Wolarsky, N., Goss, A., & Caron, B. (2020, Executive Producers). *The Crown* (Series 4, Episode 7). *Left Bank Pictures & Sony Pictures Television*. First broadcast: November 15th 2020.

Mouchenik, Y., & Fau-Vincenti, V. (2019). The Fate of Jews in Psychiatric Hospitals in Occupied Europe during the Second World War. *L'information Psychiatrique*, 95(7), 544–558.

Murthy, P., & Sekar, K. (2008). A Decade after the NHRC Quality Assurance Initiative: Current Status of Government Psychiatric Hospitals in India. *Mental Health Care and Human Rights*, 101.

NHS. (2022). *Mental Health Act Statistics Annual Figures*. https://digital.nhs.uk/ data-and-information/publications/statistical/mental-health-act-statistics-annual-figures/2021–22-annual-figures (accessed May 27th 2023).

Powell, E. (1961). Address to the National Association for Mental Health. In *Emerging Patterns for the Mental Health Services and the Public*. London: NAMH.

Scull, A. (2015). *Madness in Civilization: A Cultural History of Insanity from the Bible to Freud, from the Madhouse to Modern Medicine*. London: Thames and Hudson.

Shepherd, A., & Wright, D. (2002). Madness, Suicide and the Victorian Asylum: Attempted Self-Murder in the Age of Non-Restraint. *Medical History*, 46, 175–196.

Surrey History Centre (SHC) *Casebooks (Female) Brookwood Asylum*, 1871, Acc. 1523/3/21/2.

Taylor, B. (2014). *The Last Asylum*. London: Penguin.

Turner J., Hayward, R., Angel, K., Fulford, B., Hall, J., Millard C., & Thomson, M. (2015). The History of Mental Health Services in Modern England: Practitioner Memories and the Direction of Future Research. *Medical History*, 59(4), 599–624.

Von Bueltzingsloewen, I. (2002). The Mentally Ill Who Died of Starvation in French Psychiatric Hospitals during the German Occupation in World War II. *Vingtieme Siecle. Revue d'histoire*, 76(4), 99–115.

Wall, O. (2018). *The British Anti Psychiatrists*. London: Routledge.

Wills, C. (2021). Life Pushed Aside. *London Review of Books*, 4(12).

Wise, S. (2013). *Inconvenient People – Lunacy, Liberty and the Mad-doctors in Victorian England*. London: Vintage.

2 Anti-psychiatry
The impact of Laing, Szasz and others

This other place in a city many miles from London was in fact not called a 'hospital' at all. It had a pleasant and neutral-sounding name followed by the word 'house,' a compromise in name, though not in function, which continues in the signposting of mental health services to this day.

The original 'asylum for lunatics' had been opened in 1870, and like many others was named after the farm on whose land it was built, the word 'asylum' later replaced by the word 'hospital.' Its history was very similar to its Victorian contemporaries described in Chapter 1, and so just over a century after the hospital was built, it would be closed. As the old hospital was being run down in the 1980s, a smaller residential mental health provision was created in an annex near to the General Hospital. Mental illness was placed close to but not too close to physical illness.

This was where I was admitted in early 1985. Memories, of course, fade over time and are clouded and distorted by illness and medication. My main memories are of an L-shaped corridor downstairs with a gym, community area and offices. I remember less well the sleeping arrangements upstairs, so for the purposes of this book, I asked someone who had been a nurse there at the time to describe the living arrangements:

> *Off the corridor were single rooms. There was the Extra Care Unit which was through a locked door with a window which looked on to the corridor. At the bottom of that ward were three or four seclusion rooms – the lock ups for patients who were difficult to manage.*

We were called 'patients' then, though the terminology would change over the next 40 years.

I spent the first few nights in a small male dormitory, and I remember not sleeping because the man in the bed next to me couldn't stop crying. He was about the same age as me and a teacher in a local school. Like everyone you meet in residential mental health provision, you wonder what happened to them, how their lives panned out. But you never find out. Something which I do remember is the large number of young nurses at the hospital either in

DOI: 10.4324/9781003455042-2

training or at the very beginning of their careers, a situation which persists to this day, as we will see in Chapter 5. I remember many of them, using this phrase a lot:

There is no such thing as mental illness.

This is hard to hear when you are feeling so utterly wretched and so different from how you usually feel. When you do actually feel 'ill.' So, in this chapter, I will be exploring what was behind that phrase which was so ubiquitous at that time and in that place from the mouths of so many young nurses.

Nurse training in the 1980s was not a degree-level qualification as it is today and mental health nursing had only really begun to become a dedicated profession separate from general nursing in the late 1950s when a new experimental syllabus for mental health nurses was introduced by the General Nursing Council, though not fully implemented until 1965 (Arton, 1998). People set on a career in mental health nursing would no longer be required to sit a common preliminary examination. The syllabus would cover sociology, psychology and social psychology and students would spend some time in placements outside the hospitals in the community and shadowing a community nurse. A further new syllabus, introduced in 1982, covered psychiatry, emphasised the acquisition of interpersonal skills and indicated that nurses would no longer train exclusively to work in an institution. Question 1 of the final state examination for mental health nurses, set by the General Nursing Council for England and Wales and sat on Tuesday, 1 June 1982, gives an indication of the culture of the time:

Institutionalisation begins upon admission to hospital.

(a) Describe how the process of admission may confirm and re-enforce the 'patient role.'
(b) How should the nurse assist patients to maintain their self-identity during the admission period and subsequent care?

This question had echoes of the large-scale closures of the old 'asylums' which were underway by the mid-1980s, and also of a movement in psychiatry which had flourished more than a decade earlier, but whose influence persisted then and persists today: 'anti-psychiatry.'

Wall (2016) sketches the background of the 'anti-psychiatry' movement to the 1960s – the 'decade of revolutions . . . when The West was shaken by waves of protest from civil rights marches in the United States, to anti – Vietnam War demonstrations across Europe, to the May Days in France' (p. 3). This was not only about rising up against old institutions, but also against old ideas and old definitions, and psychiatry itself could not escape this process. Wall traces the origins of these shifts in social and political attitudes to the memory of the Second World War. The trauma of the concentration camps was an 'assault on humanity' (p. 131), and liberation from the old ways in so many areas was 'the restoration of humanity in a dehumanised culture' (p. 122).

It is no coincidence then that the anti-psychiatry movement was at its most influential just as the drive to close the large asylums was gaining ground and many of the same actors straddled both movements. It was no longer enough simply to see beyond the crumbling old hospitals: the anti-psychiatrics also 'vociferously abandoned institutional psychiatry' (p. 2) and the very meaning of mental illness was up for question as well.

There is some debate about who actually first coined the phrase 'no such thing as mental illness,' but the prime movers in anti-psychiatry were mostly, and perhaps curiously, psychiatrists: Thomas Szasz born in 1920 in Hungary; Ervin Goffman, an American-Canadian Sociologist born in 1922; Ronald David ('R.D.') Laing born in 1927 in Glasgow, and David Cooper born in 1931 in South Africa. There were, and still are, others of course and their works and theories have been widely read, critiqued, compared and contrasted by practitioners and academics, some of whom are cited in this chapter, but it is worth briefly summarising here what bound them all together as 'anti-psychiatrists.'

The ideas behind the movement were 'borrowed from a wide variety of writers in different disciplines' (Wall, 2016, p. 19), including Franco Basaglia, whose influence on the closure of the asylums in Italy will be seen in Chapter 4, and also the French surrealist Andre Breton and existentialist writers such as Jean-Paul Sartre. The 'idea of existential reality is central to much of the anti-psychiatric literature' (p. 123), especially in the 'gap between the reality of the world as articulated by society and the way a person experiences it himself' (p. 123). In his article 'The Rise and Fall of Anti-psychiatry' (1995), Nasser states that it was the French psychologist Jacques Lacan (1901–1981) who was 'probably the first to glorify madness and regard it as the path to freedom' (p. 743) in his *Propos sur la causalité psychique* (1947) and Laing said much the same thing in *The Politics of Experience* (1967), but it was Szasz who arguably was the first to reject the idea of mental illness altogether saying that 'the mind cannot be diseased as it is not an organ of the body' (p. 745). Mental illness, then, does not really exist or at least does not exist to anything like the extent people were being led to believe and mental illnesses 'cannot legitimately be categorised as diseases' (Benning, 2016, p. 292).

Szasz did not deny that humans have difficulties and that there is real suffering in these difficulties but preferred to conceptualise them not as mental illnesses, but as 'problems in living' (Benning, 2016 p. 292), regarding mental illness as a 'construct misappropriating medical concepts in order to control people whose behaviour was regarded as alarming or offensive' (Turner et al., 2015, p. 617):

[T]hat physicians and patients insist that psychotherapy *is* medical treatment is no more surprising than that Medieval Catholic priests insisted that ceremonial wine *is* human blood.

(Szasz, 1979, p. 190)

Szasz argued that individuals are 'always responsible for their conduct' (Benning, 2016, p. 293) and Laing (1967) asserted that 'without exception the experience and behaviours that get labelled schizophrenic are a special strategy that a person invents in order to live in an unliveable situation' (p. 95). More widely 'the contradictions and confusions 'internalised' by the individual must be looked at in their larger social contexts' (p. 96)

Those social contexts resided in the political upheavals of the time, as well as in the family unit, and for the anti-psychiatrists, the emotional difficulties experienced by people had causes linked to oppression and inequality, with psychiatry no more than a political power play aimed at keeping people enslaved. Laing (1967) expressed it like this:

> There is no such 'condition' as 'schizophrenia,' but the label is a social fact and the social fact a political event. . . . This political event . . . is a social prescription that rationalises a set of social actions whereby the labelled person is annexed by others.
>
> (p. 95)

Goffman (1961) called both the medical model and mental hospitals themselves 'vicissitudes of the tinkering trades' (p. 321) and Cooper saw 'modern psychiatry as a pseudo-science which grew hand in hand with capitalism as society's repressive device' (Nasser, 1995, p. 744) with conditions which are now categorised as 'illness' such as schizophrenia seen as a sane response to an insane environment created, largely, by capitalism or by a dysfunctional family unit. As a psychiatrist, it was Laing's job to look beyond behaviours, reject medical diagnosis and explore dispassionately the social and political background:

> I have difficulty in actually discovering the 'signs and symptoms' of psychosis in persons I am interviewing. 'To see 'signs' of 'disease' is not to see neutrally.
>
> (Laing, 1960, p. 32)

For Goffman (1961), 'the patient's life is regulated and ordered according to a disciplinarian system developed for the management by a small staff of a large number of inmates' (p. 361), and given a broader audience by Ken Kesey just a year later in his novel *One Flew over the Cuckoo's Nest*, which had a significant impact on its readers' views of mental illness, an impact which would increase with the release of the film version in 1975:

> Not in the hospital to get fixed, but to stop them walking around the streets giving the product a bad name.
>
> (Kesey, 1962, p. 14)

The irony then for Goffman was that although the patient is made into a 'serviceable object . . . so little service is available once this is done' (Goffman, 1961, p. 379). We will see later in the book that this is an issue which is as relevant in mental health provision today as it was to the anti-psychiatrists in the 1960s.

This then may explain why I heard the phrase 'no such thing as mental illness' so often in that setting back in 1985, usually from the nurses but also in ward rounds from the consultant psychiatrist, a man who seemed to hold sway in this place with unusual power and who was talked of with awe by many of the young nurses, though less so by the old hands. It seems unlikely that in 1985 and employed as a consultant by the NHS he would have called himself an 'anti-psychiatrist,' but what he was though was someone who embraced a therapeutic approach related to anti-psychiatry: Gestalt therapy.

Gestalt therapy and the anti-psychiatry movement both had their philosophical roots in humanistic psychology (Moss, 2001). The Austro-German philosopher Edmund Husserl (1859–1938) had called for a phenomenological approach in both philosophy and psychology with his cry of returning 'to the things themselves' (Husserl, 1970) and his emphasis on the intentionality of human mental activity. French philosopher Maurice Merleau-Ponty (1908–1961) reinforced this by noting that no human behaviour can be separated from its environment, context and situation, a concept of course also espoused by the anti-psychiatrists. 'Gestalt' is a German word loosely translated by the English phrase 'whole shape' and Gestalt therapy is about the whole person as an individual capable of acting with agency and intention.

It was the German psychiatrist Fritz Perls (1893–1970) and his wife the psychologist Laura Perls (1905–1990), who, dissatisfied with Freudian psychotherapy, channelled these and their own existential ideas into a radical new humanistic therapy, with ideas about the self and self-awareness at its core. Perls' book *Gestalt Therapy* was published in 1951 and the first Gestalt Institute was established in New York in the early 1950s.

One of the more controversial aspects of Gestalt therapy (Mann, 2010) lies in 'carefully graded experimentation and challenge in therapy' (p. 127). The therapist and their client create a situation that will challenge the client's fixed mindsets and outdated ways of being. Handled with care, this Gestalt approach can lead to metamorphosis and recovery. This brings us back to that consultant psychiatrist.

As I have said before, this book is not a memoir. My own experiences with in-patient mental health care are only drawn upon to shed light on policy and practice. The 'lived experience' of the title is largely my own, and so it must always be borne in mind that memory, my own memory perhaps in particular, can be fickle and uncertain, especially when recalling uncomfortable events. My experiences with this consultant are now nearly 40 years ago, and so I turned to that former nurse from that hospital, and their memories of him are kinder than my own:

> *I didn't dislike him. In ward rounds he was always fairly gentle, doggedly against ECT and encouraged us student nurses to have their say.*

Nevertheless, these are three of my own encounters with him which I remember most vividly:

1) I am in his office. It is what is known as a 'ward round' where, usually weekly, there is a review of your case with a team of staff. My memory though is of being alone with the consultant. 'How are you feeling?,' he asks. 'I feel like shit,' I reply. 'I think everyone thinks I am a shit as well.' 'Well, perhaps you have always been a little shit?,' he suggests.
2) I meet him in a corridor. Now I know no one likes to be asked a question at work in the corridor but when I ask him: 'Can I speak to you?,' he says: 'Fuck off.'
3) I have absconded but don't get far and am picked up by two kindly policemen and sat in the back of their car. They have a conversation over their radio with the consultant. 'What did he say?,' I ask. 'He said: "you can bloody well keep him." '

I can only assume that this was him using the 'challenge' technique of Gestalt therapy, though, as Mann (2010) points out, 'challenging a client does not necessarily mean vigorous confrontation or the client getting into some strong emotion' (p. 127). In my case, it did not lead to metamorphosis or recovery.

Gestalt therapy is still a valid and respected part of the cannon of talking therapies around the world. I have spoken to people who have benefitted from it enormously and a few who found it overly harsh and challenging. It has survived the shifting sands of policy and practice into the 21st century and will probably do so for a long time to come.

The anti-psychiatry movement had less happy outcomes, and the influence of Laing, Szasz and others came to be seen as 'more to do with political and professional pragmatism than with the scientific validity or practical utility of their findings' (Jack, 1998, p. 1). Less kindly, as Benning (2016) reminds us, 'there is a reality and suffering attached to mental illness, to psychological dysfunction, that Szasz's writings simply fail to acknowledge' (p. 294). Lieberman (2004) is even less forgiving: 'I think Szasz trivializes devastating malfunction – serious mental illness – by dismissing such patients as attention seekers, imposters, and so forth.' Wall (2016) charts the start of this general disillusion with anti-psychiatry to 1969 when 'even those sections of mainstream psychiatry who had been sympathetic to the idea . . . turned against it' (p. 78).

It was a controversial movement, but 'it is naïve to assume that the anti-psychiatry movement has little or no impact on the way psychiatry is conceived and practiced today' (Nasser p. 745) and, as we will see in Chapter 5, it was still hovering around in 2020 and it certainly helped to popularise the critique of psychiatry as a disciplinary practice, to open public debates on the role of psychiatry in society and to further destabilise the already shaky social position of the mental hospital. In part, it also further paved the way for the birth of the Service Users' Movements (Wall, 2018 p. 8) such as the Patient Advice and Liaison Service (PALS) which is very much alive within the NHS in England today as are many charities which support people in in-patient settings.

Neither David Cooper nor R.D. Laing, two of the chief actors in the movement, took part in the continuing debates over 'anti-psychiatry' in the ensuing decades (Wall, 2016). Cooper moved to Argentina, drank heavily, experimented with drugs and died of a heart attack in 1985 at the age of 54. Laing wrote poetry and persisted with his psychiatric work, but in 1986 the General Medical Council began an investigation into him after complaints that he had been drunk and abusive during therapy sessions. In 1987, he was invited to withdraw his name from the medical register. He died of a heart attack while playing tennis in St Tropez in 1989 at the age of 62.

And me . . . ?

I was discharged with no backup from one NHS in-patient provision in the process of change, and a few days later was admitted to a place at the other end of the country, a place itself at the crossroads of policy and practice, a place I had first visited ten years before in my delivery van, a place where my experience of in-patient mental health care would be very different indeed . . . .

References

Arton, M. (1998). *The Professionalism of Mental Health Nursing in Britain*, A Dissertation Submitted for the Degree of Doctor of Philosophy. History of Medicine, University College London.

Benning, T. (2016). No Such Thing as Mental Illness? Critical Reflections on the Major Ideas and Legacy of Thomas Szasz. *BJPsych Bulletin*, 40(6), 292–295.

Goffman, E. (1961). *Asylums: Essays on the Social Situation of Mental Patients and Other Inmates*. Chicago: Aldine Publisher, Co.

Husserl, E. (1970). *Logical Investigations Volume 1*. London: Routledge and Kegan Paul.

Jack, R. (1998). Institutions in Community Care. In Jack, R. (Ed.), *Residential versus Community Care – The Role of Institutions in Welfare Provision*. London: MacMillan Press.

Kesey, K. (1962). *One Flew Over the Cuckoos Nest*. London: Penguin Books.

Laing, R.D. (1960). *The Divided Self: An Existential Study in Sanity and Madness*. Harmondsworth: Penguin.

Laing, R.D. (1967). *The Politics of Experience*. Harmondsworth: Penguin.

Lieberman, E.J. (2004) Pharmacracy or Phantom. In Schaler, J.A. (Ed.), *Szasz Under Fire: The Psychiatric Abolitionist Faces His Critics*, pp. 225–241. Chicago: Open Court.

Mann, D. (2010). *Gestalt Therapy: 100 Key Points and References*. London: Routledge.

Moss, D. (2001). The Roots and Genealogy of Humanistic Psychology. In *The Handbook of Humanistic Psychology: Leading Edges in Theory, Research, and Practice*, pp. 5–20. Thousand Oaks: Sage Publications.

Nasser, M. (1995). The Rise and Fall of Anti-psychiatry. *Psychiatric Bulletin of the Royal College of Psychiatrists*, 19(12), 743–746. https://doi.org/10.1192/pb.19.12.743

Szasz, T. (1979). *The Myth of Psychotherapy: Mental Healing as Religion, Rhetoric and Repression*. Oxford: Oxford University Press.

Turner, J., Hayward, R., Angel, K., Fulford, B., Hall, J., Millard, C., & Thomson, M. (2015). The History of Mental Health Services in Modern England: Practitioner Memories and the Direction of Future Research. *Medical History*, 59(4), 599–624. https://doi.org/10.1017/mdh.2015.48.

Wall, O. (2018). *The British Anti Psychiatrists*. London: Routledge.

3 The last years of the asylums

Return to Netherne Hospital

By 1985, most of the old Victorian asylums were still around and more or less functioning, though all were being wound down: some of their patients were being moved on, and many of their buildings were already standing empty. One such was Netherne Hospital in Coulsdon Surrey, where I had delivered outpatient work less than ten years before. It was not properly 'Victorian' at all because although it had been conceived in the last years of Queen Victoria's reign, it didn't open till eight years after her death and was one of the last institutions of its type to be built in the UK (McCrae & Nolan, 2016). It had been built on a hill to the east of the main London to Brighton railway line on extensive farmland and accessed via a long road which meandered up through fields and woods. I am grateful to Clair Wills in her excellent article on Netherne, 'Life Pushed Aside,' in *The London Review of Books* (2021) for quoting John Betjeman's poem 'Croydon' as providing an image of the landscape around the hospital in the 1930s and one which still held true in 1985:

> Boys together in Coulsdon woodlands/Bramble berried and steep.
>
> (Betjeman, 1970)

In the first 30 years or so of its existence, Netherne functioned very much like all the other great asylums as a place of confinement and custody, though in some respects its original design hinted at its future as a more forgiving and humane place with a number of separate smaller 'villas' built within the spacious grounds and an admissions unit built away from the main hospital block. This was a decidedly modern development as in most of the other hospitals admissions were 'received at the business end of a daunting edifice' (McRae and Nolan, 216, p. 78). It was also more or less self-sufficient:

> Netherne had its own vegetable and dairy farm (with labour provided by the patients), a bakery, kitchens, laundry, carpentry and light engineering workshops, a printing press, chapel, library, cinema, dance hall, orchestra, choir, sport facilities and an amateur dramatic society.
>
> (Wills, 2021, p. 23)

DOI: 10.4324/9781003455042-3

After the Second World War, the arrival of two key modernising superin-tendents and an influential artist moved Netherne towards becoming such a model of good therapeutic practice that it was visited by three Health Secre-taries and Eleanor Roosevelt, the widow of the US wartime leader Franklin.

Eric Cunningham-Dax (1908–2008) was Physician Superintendent at Netherne from 1946 to 1951 when he emigrated to New Zealand and was replaced by Dr Rudolf Freudenberg (1908–1983), who remained in post till his retirement in 1973. Both men appreciated the importance of social factors in mental health, but also saw the key role of the in-patient hospital in the treatment of mental illness. Freudenberg disagreed with Enoch Powell. He felt strongly that outcomes for patients would be bettered not by demolishing the old asylums but by making changes within them. Freudenberg worked at Netherne alongside the psychiatrist and later pioneer in the field of autism studies, Dr Lorna Wing, and they went on to reduce overcrowding, provide more occupation and improve the clothing, care and attention received by the patients, with Netherne becoming one of the first hospitals to employ a soci-ologist (McCrae & Nolan, 2016).

Freudenberg also took the bold step of unlocking many of the wards and removing the fences which surrounded them, a move which attracted world-wide coverage in the press. In 1956, he supervised a sociological study carried out by MS Folkard into the impact on aggression of opening previously closed wards. In a conclusion that echoes current issues, which will be discussed in later chapters, Folkard wrote:

> The evidence would seem to suggest that the unlocking of the door was one factor in helping to reduce the amount of aggression on the ward, but this by itself is not a complete solution to the problem . . . other events, such as changes amongst the nurses on the ward can produce an increase in the amount of disturbance.
>
> (1959, p. 139)

During his tenure at the hospital, Cunningham-Dax had brought in an artist, Edward Adamson (1911–1996), to work with patients. Freudenberg cham-pioned Adamson's work at the hospital and by the late 1950s, Netherne had become a pioneer and world leader in the use of art as therapy. Active at Netherne from 1946 to 1981, Adamson's patients produced thousands of paintings, sculptures and other works and the vast 'Adamson Collection' is now held at the Wellcome Archive at Euston in London.

Shortly after he gave his 'Water Towers' speech in March 1961, Enoch Powell made his one and only visit to Netherne Hospital. He will have seen the imposing water tower and the tall chimney but surely didn't stay long enough to take in the many innovations in therapeutic care that Cunningham-Dax, Freudenberg, Wing, Adamson and others had introduced. One assumes he must have met Dr Freudenberg, but no record of any such meeting exists. It must have been a very remarkable encounter indeed: the gentle hospital doctor who had fled Hitler's Germany in 1934 and was described in his obituary as 'an extremely modest man who cloaked his warm and humorous sympathy with shy formality' (Godard, 1983) in the same room as the orator and Conservative politician who just a few years later would make his notorious 'Rivers of Blood' speech criticising the Race Relations Bill (1968) which set out to promote harmonious community relations in the UK. Within months of Powell's visit to Netherne, the poultry farm was closed, and next to go was the main farm, despite the fact that the hospital had just purchased a state-of-the-art milking parlour for its cows (Frogley & Welch, 1993). By 1965, Netherne had lost its own management committee and came under the wing of Redhill General Hospital. In the ensuing years, the shoemakers' shop, tailors' shop and the upholstery department would all close down. The hospital's own fire brigade, which had employed non-nursing staff and patients together for over 50 years, staggered on till 1986, when it was finally disbanded.

So when I was driven up that long winding road in the early spring of 1985, Netherne was a shadow of its former self. The vast main building with its single curving corridor reputed to be nearly a third of a mile long was still in use, and many of the 20 or more wards off this corridor were still occupied, but some of the villas which had accommodated smaller communities of patients were shuttered. The chapel and concert hall stood empty. There were about 700 patient beds left, down from a peak of over 2,000 a couple of decades before.

I was soon to find out though that within the still working hospital, the staff were striving to hang on to the best of a fading system, a system dedicated not to confinement but to 'moral treatment,' to the best of what Freudenberg, Adamson and others had put in place even though it was being dismantled around them. I was to be in John Reid House, a large two-storeyed building set a hundred yards or so from the main hospital with beds for maybe 30 patients but also its own rehabilitation unit and day hospital. Like the rest of the hospital, John Reid House was at the crossroads of the old and the new: the old was the vast imposing hospital itself with its acres of grounds. The new was its smaller scale, and the acceptance that if you were in there, you wouldn't be for long. I never felt the slightest chance of becoming institutionalised, though as we will see a little later, I would come across, in a far corner of the hospital, an extreme case of institutionalisation.

The consultant psychiatrist who admitted me put it like this: *We'll sort you out. A few weeks in here, medication, exercise, a few activities, maybe even a little job. You'll feel better soon.* I didn't believe him, but as it turned out, he was right.

I was very ill when I arrived at Netherne, and my memory of those first couple of weeks is unclear. I spent the first few nights in a 'suicide watch' ward which was a small dormitory separated from the observation room by a wall of glass. I was then given my own room with a large window overlooking the open countryside, though I didn't take much notice at the time. It was a small and simple bedroom: a wooden desk, a chair, a bedside table. A crucifix and one or two other pictures on the wall. As we will see in Chapter 5, the issue of 'ligature points' in bedrooms would be far more rigorously addressed by 2020. Here we were simply discouraged from going up to our rooms during the day.

Exactly as the consultant who admitted me had said, I was given medication – a lot of medication: I think 15 pills a day. I don't remember all the names, but there was less choice back then and I think only one of them was actually meant to address my 'nervous disorder,' the rather quaint term used on my hospital record. The others were largely to address the side effects of the main medication, side effects which included dry mouth, dizziness, weight gain and, only discovered years later, an ectopic heartbeat.

It was the 'activity' the consultant promised me which I think contributed as much to my recovery as all the pills. I was tasked with painting the metal frame of an old pagoda in the grounds, a task I shared with a woman, herself an artist, who spoke so rarely, and then so quietly that we completed the task in a sort of meditative and companionable silence. Physical activity arrived at the door of my room in the middle of one morning in the shape of a young student nurse carrying a pair of what were then called 'plimsoles.' He had been reading my notes and seen that before I became ill, before I slumped into inactivity and chain smoking, I had been quite sporty and had enjoyed running. He didn't force me, but he suggested politely that perhaps we could go for a run together. That first one was hard – and short. I was not a willing participant, but after that he turned up every morning, and every morning we ran a little further around the grounds, alongside fields, through the trees. His name, I think, was Graham, and I will never be able to thank him enough. Then there was the art.

Edward Adamson had only retired from Netherne a few years before my admission, and his presence was still there in the hospital's many large art rooms. Almost every day a few of us would shuffle into one of these – a room full of light from the tall windows and on the walls paintings, drawings and collages made by patients long discharged or dead. We would sit where we wanted – at a table, an easel or an armchair – drink tea, smoke, and talk – to each other a bit but mainly with the art therapist, who listened. We were never told what to do or make and sometimes we did nothing at all, but often we would paint a little or cut out shapes and stick them on paper, or mess around with charcoal. Adamson believed that the process of making art could itself be therapeutic and that art had the ability to provide a way of communicating (Noble & Hackett, 2023). In this spirit, the art therapist at Netherne in 1985 would look, and sometimes comment very softly but never judgementally, and always listen. Like Graham, he was in the right job, doing the right thing, at the right time, and in retrospect, nearly 40 years later, I can see that there was a kind of gentle alchemy going on in that room. I couldn't say with any certainty, even today, what exactly 'art therapy' is or how it works, and it takes a Masters' Degree to become an art therapist, but it was what we were doing, and it was right.

And then, suddenly, one day in May 1985, the last thing that the consultant had promised me came about. I woke up, but on this morning I didn't pull the sheets over my head wanting it all just to go away whilst I waited for Graham's knock on the door. Instead, I got up and walked to the window. The sun was shining on the most beautiful chestnut tree, in fact the most beautiful tree, I had ever seen. It had been there all along of course, but now the catastrophic thoughts, the anxieties, the terrible images which had been turning in my head for six months had stilled. I had stilled. I was able to look at that tree, focus on that tree alone and actually see it. I can still see it now.

That same day I noticed for the first time an old record player in the corner of the patients' lounge, beside it a few long-playing records. I put one of them on the turntable. It was Bob Dylan's *Blood on the Tracks* and, like seeing the tree, it was as if I was hearing it for the first time – those deep base notes and the poetry in the lyrics. Later that evening I sat in the lounge and watched a film on the old black and white television in the corner. It was Clint Eastwood's 1971 thriller *Play Misty for Me*, and I sat there and watched it all the way through. It was the first time I had sat still for more than a minute or two for six months, the first time I had watched anything on the TV all the way through. I had, literally, come back to my senses.

I was still fragile of course and spent a further two months or so as an in-patient in Netherne as well as the rest of that year as a day patient as the medication was gradually reduced and phased out, but in that spring of 1985 my reawakened gaze would notice much about this old asylum in the last years of its life.

John Reid House was a temporary home for people from all backgrounds and circumstances: there were Fleet Street print workers whose mental health had been shattered by their working conditions and by the beginning of the end of their industry before the Wapping disputes the following year; there were teachers, a socialite, a man who spoke in a dialect not un-similar to Shakespearean English, a woman who had been engaged for ten years to a man who would never agree on a wedding date and there was 'Michael,' who became my friend, a man who had lost his mind playing his violin on the streets of Berlin. We were a community of sorts, made tea for each other in the communal kitchen, shared cigarettes, watched TV together and even put on a play. I have no recollection of what it was about, but I do remember that one of the cast members insisted on wearing the grey top hat he never took off on the ward, and the play was all the better for it.

I don't remember much about the food, except for tapioca, which I would meet again in 2020, but I do remember that meals were taken in quite a formal dining room at tables with tablecloths for five or six people. Other than the occasional bowl of porridge thrown against the wall, I don't remember much disruption to mealtimes. At Netherne everyone, even the nurses, seemed to smoke, possibly even during meals. We know from a number of studies that smoking rates among people with a mental health condition are disproportionately higher than average national smoking rates across the world, with the highest levels of smoking found in psychiatric in-patients (Pooja & Driscoll, 2020), and we will see later on in this book that smoking in in-patient mental health units has now become a literal battleground, with casualties on all sides.

The nurses and other staff at the hospital were from diverse backgrounds and cultures. Recruitment had always been a problem in mental health services because of relatively low rates of pay and a perception that working conditions were worse than in general nursing. After the Second World War, 'hospital managers in the south of England increasingly looked across the Irish Sea' (Mcrae and Nolan, p. 207), and then further afield to the West Indies and former colonies and the staff at Netherne reflected that, with in particular a very large number of Irish nurses. Many of these had come across a decade earlier with their families to help construct the M25 motorway, which was close by, and had stayed on to build their own careers in the NHS.

Beyond John Reid House, what went on in other parts of the hospital was also a mix of the old and the new. The floor of the endless corridor which curved through the main building was always being mopped and polished, sometimes by cleaners but also by patients. Other patients walked up and down it, or sat against the walls, some barefoot, occasionally scarcely clothed. The wards behind the doors were places of mystery. Some of the remaining villas in the grounds had become rehabilitation units, preparing people for the inevitable step back into the community. This rehabilitation and resettlement work had been another initiative pioneered in 1957 by Dr Freudenberg who saw the importance of preparing patients for life outside the hospital and this ethos continued into the 1980s with programmes established to teach patients techniques of how to behave during job interviews, and a Clerical Intensive Therapy Organisation offering training in office skills. This ethos, whilst establishing Netherne as a forerunner in the development of community care, would also contribute to the demise of the hospital itself.

A few of these remaining villas though were sinister places and around them swirled rumour and innuendo about who they were for and what went on in them, but if there were issues with restraint and confinement, even abuse, they were out of sight. A resident from one of them did occasionally come over to play table tennis with us. He was a giant man with latent aggression simmering under his every word and gesture. The bats and balls didn't last long. But he was also a talented artist who drew intricate designs for space rockets, some of which, with the support of the hospital staff, he would send to NASA in America.

In Netherne Hospital, I think I mostly felt safe. I was though sexually assaulted in John Reid House, by a fellow patient: the one I earlier called, possibly unjustly, 'the socialite.' She forced me into an unlocked cupboard and pressed herself against me, pulling at my clothes, but I was able to make my escape. I can't remember if I reported this, but a few hours later we were both playing cards with other patients in the lounge.

In the asylum system as it had existed for more than a century, and particularly with the influence of therapeutic communities such as The York Retreat and Geel in Belgium, 'work by patients was a central content' (Johnson & Walmsley, 2010, p. 103). So just a day or two before I woke up and noticed the chestnut tree, I had started the other thing the consultant had promised me: 'a little job,' and a paid one at that: I helped out at what was known then as a 'psycho-geriatric' ward on the far side of the grounds beyond the cricket pitch. My working hours were 10 a.m. to 12 noon and 2 p.m. to 4 p.m. I made tea, chatted to the patients and was given the job of sorting through the bags of clean washing which would arrive every morning, pairing up the socks and putting them in drawers. This was the first real job of any kind I had been able to do for six months. It was something I could do, and it was a building block for my return to the workplace nearly a year later.

The patients on this ward were generally over the age of around 65 and were living with dementia in its various forms, though for one or two the disease had caught them much younger and a lady of about 50 would in occasional moments of lucidity sob uncontrollably at her fate. They were a quirky and sometimes challenging group, some of whom who had been abandoned by their families, but they were loved and cared for by the staff. One man enjoyed urinating in the pot plants which adorned the wards, but no one got angry with him, and the plants were not locked away. If he was seen heading towards a pot and undoing his flies, he was simply steered gently towards the toilet.

I enjoyed my 'little job' and the routine and simple tasks undoubtedly helped in my recovery. What is more, every Friday I would queue up at a window inside the main hospital where I would be given my pay, just a few pounds, in a small brown envelope. What did I spend it on? I don't really remember. Cigarettes maybe, though by then I barely needed them. Sweets? A newspaper? The little things of a normal life.

The topic of 'institutionalisation' – what it is or isn't – is a recurrent theme in this book, but in that psycho-geriatric ward I saw it, and I understood all too clearly what it was. There was a man on the ward who was 90 years old. I know that because one of the nurses told me he had been born in 1895, but that was almost all anyone knew about him. What records there were showed that he had stolen a milk bottle when he was ten years old, which had led him being admitted to Netherne and rejected by his family, and there he had stayed for the rest of his life. He hadn't fought in the Great War, he hadn't had a job or lost it in the Great Depression, he hadn't voted, he hadn't married or had a family, he hadn't joined the Home Guard or retired with a carriage clock. He hadn't seen the momentous events of the 1960s or had an opinion about

Margaret Thatcher. He hadn't done any of things in life which mark us, and that must have been why his face had no wrinkles, the skin almost as smooth as it must have been when he stole that milk bottle. A few years later, he would have been buried in Netherne's own cemetery alongside all those who had no other final resting place or family to mourn them.

In 1990, the English actress Dame Judi Dench, alongside her husband Michael Williams, were cast in a TV play called *Can You Hear Me Thinking?*, and part of the filming took place at Netherne, which by then was down to its last 200 or so patients. It was an experience they would never forget, and later Dame Judi would the following in her Foreword to Frogley and Welch's *A Pictorial History of Netherne* (1992):

> Reading this history of the hospital, one thing stands out – the devotion to not only the health but the welfare of its patients, despite at times, chronic overcrowding, and lack of funds and staff. Those who could be cured were returned to the community, though the door was always open should things become too difficult. For those who were not able to cope in the outside world, Netherne was a home.
>
> The dictionary defines 'asylum' as a 'place of sanctuary, a refuge.' Netherne offered not only a refuge but hope to many during its history.

That is what Netherne had offered me: a sanctuary, a place of refuge where I could begin to rebuild my life, which I did more or less successfully, until more than 30 years later I entered the dark tunnel of mental illness again. It offered the same to many people, just as down the road Cane Hill had offered a more long-term refuge to those Polish airmen. It has even been said (Turner et al., 2015) that 'in spite of Enoch Powell's apocalyptic threats' (p. 207) 20 years before, the 1980s was the best time that the mental hospitals ever had. Money wasn't flowing freely, but there was more than there had been, numbers of patients were falling, while the staff numbers were being preserved because the new acute psychiatric units being created in general hospitals had not yet started 'luring talented nurses from the mental institutions' (McCrae and Nolan, p. 198). The standard of nursing care was possibly as good as it had been for years. There was also, in most cases, enough money to make the old accommodation certainly tolerable, if not quite satisfactory, but the system it belonged to – the 'asylum system' – kept that smooth-faced old man and many others too long and stopped them from getting on with their own lives in a wider community. As Clair Wills put it at the end of her 2021 article 'Lives Pushed Aside' in *The London Review of Books:*

> Despite the sunlit grounds and the airy wards and the seemingly porous border between the inside and the outside of the institution, you could still be buried alive there.

(p. 29)

My own experience in Netherne in 1985 was generally speaking positive, and maybe that was because I was there in that between time, the early 1980s, when there were still those precious commodities: time, space and money. I am not though an apologist for the old 'asylums,' and this book is not proposing a return to the old asylum system. Some terrible things went on within those stark walls: some witnessed, some documented, but many others unrecorded except by the scars on the minds and bodies of those who suffered. But terrible things continue to go on within in-patient care today. We have not solved the problem by demolishing the asylums, but demolish them we did, and we moved on to a system which, superficially at least, seemed altogether new and different.

References

Betjeman, J. (1970). *John Betjeman's Collected Poems, Enlarged Edition.* London: John Murray.

Folkard, M. (1959). *A Sociological Contribution to the Understanding of Aggression and Its Treatment Based upon Social Research Performed at Netherne Hospital, Coulsdon, Surrey.* Coulsdon: Netherne Monographs.

Frogley, G., & Welch, J. (1993). *A Pictorial History of Netherne.* Redhill: East Surrey Health Authority.

Godard, P. (1983). *Rudolf Karl Freudenberg, Formerly Physician Superintendent, Netherne Hospital, Coulsdon, Surrey.* Cambridge: Cambridge University Press.

Johnson, K., Walmsley, J., with Wolfe, M. (2010). *People with Intellectual Disabilities – Towards a Good Life?* Bristol: The Policy Press.

McCrae, N., & Nolan, P. (2016). *The Story of Nursing in British Mental Hospitals – Echoes from the Corridors.* London: Routledge.

Noble, J., & Hackett S. (2023). Art Therapy in Acute Inpatient Care. *International Journal of Art Therapy.* https://doi.org/10.1080/17454832.2023.2175003.

Pooja, P., & Driscoll R. (2020). 'Quit during COVID-19' – Staying Smokefree in Mental Health In-patient Settings. *Ecancer 2020*, 14th ed, p. 102. www.ecancer.org; https://doi.org/10.3332/ecancer.2020.ed102

Powell, E. (1961). Address to the National Association for Mental Health. In *Emerging Patterns for the Mental Health Services and the Public.* London: NAMH.

Turner J., Hayward, R., Angel, K., Fulford, B., Hall, J., Millard C., & Thomson, M. (2015). The History of Mental Health Services in Modern England: Practitioner Memories and the Direction of Future Research. *Medical History*, 59(4), 599–624.

Wills, C. (2021). Life Pushed Aside. *London Review of Books*, 43(12).

4 Exclusion or inclusion

Out of the hospitals and into the community

Netherne Hospital wasn't so much demolished as recycled, but first the remaining patients had to be recycled too. In 1988, there were just 616 of them left. By 1993, this number had fallen to 150 and on Tuesday, 9 August 1994, the last 12 residents were moved on. They were each presented with copies of a painting of the old hospital. The local paper *The Mirror* sent a photographer along and took a photo of 12 of them linking arms and apparently walking purposefully away from their old home. They were moved mostly to smaller units or houses in nearby towns whilst those with more serious illnesses were transferred to a new ward at the local General Hospital, the type of provision which would become the norm over the next 30 years. The article in *The Mirror* reassures its readers that 'the care, treatment and rehabilitation the hospital once provided is now provided under the Care in the Community programme' (Gumb, 1994) and quotes Sally Smith, chief executive of the NHS Watchdog the Community Health Council:

> [A] wide range of alternative facilities have been developed to meet people's needs . . . and the local population has its part to play in recognising that it is right for care to be provided in the local community rather than in the large asylums.

Also present at the little ceremony was local Conservative MP Sir George Gardiner who commented hopefully:

> When former patients are discharged, it is very important that they are welcomed by the community.

One small group of the last residents to leave (McCrae & Nolan, 2016) were housed in a care home with a 100-foot garden surrounded by trees where they used to sit 'in varying states of dress away from prying eyes' (p. 275). This privacy was appreciated by all. Sadly, it wasn't long before a four-storey apartment block was built next door and with their garden now overlooked, the residents retreated inside, but at least indoors there was some familiarity

DOI: 10.4324/9781003455042-4

with their former home, as the lounge was still called the 'day room' and their bedside cabinets 'lockers.'

The 178 acres of the Netherne Hospital Estate along with the old hospital buildings and more than 30 houses were put up for sale in May 1994 by competitive tender by the Secretary of State for Health. The sale was delayed because the Disused Burial Grounds Act (1898) stipulated that no land could be used for any other purpose within 100 years of the last interment in a cemetery, which meant that the cemetery at Netherne, resting place of 1,300 former patients, stood in the way of progress. Nevertheless, four tenders were received, and in 1995 the site was sold to a local property developer.

The developer's plans for the Netherne site were for 430 houses, including a retirement complex, a nursing home, a business centre, a shop, a public house with restaurant and recreational open space. Bricks from the demolished hospital would be recycled to use in the new development. We will visit what is now known as 'Netherne Village' at the end of Chapter 7 to see what happened to these ambitious plans for a sustainable community.

All over the UK the old asylums were being re-developed or left to fall into ruin – which prompted the campaigning organisation SAVE Britain's Heritage to suggest that not since the Beeching Report of 1962 led to decommissioning of so much of the railway infrastructure has so large a slice of the nation's public architectural heritage been made redundant (SAVE, 1995). Korman (1991) found that the 'institutions were created very much more rapidly than we were able to close them' (p. 12) and research by The Kings Fund in 2015 showed that many of them were not sold until many years after closure. Pace was similarly slow in other parts of the world, though Italy had bucked the trend a little by passing 'Basaglia's Law' in 1978, named after the eminent psychiatrist Franco Basaglia who was heavily influenced by Cooper, Goffman and others. The law banned all future admissions to mental hospitals and thereafter Italy embarked on a rapid programme of closures. The vast San Clemente asylum for women outside Venice was abandoned and became a stray cats' home.

In the United States, closures followed a similar pattern but were possibly driven even more by the harsh economic climate, the shortening of the working week and higher wages (Scull, 2015). In Massachusetts, Milton Greenblatt, commissioner of mental health, said: 'in a sense, our backs are against the wall. It's phase out before we go bankrupt' (ibid., p. 370). Many of the larger asylums in the United States lay empty and crumbling for decades (Scull, 2015). France, Germany, Sweden and Denmark were a little slower largely because mental hospital populations had increased during the 1970s though 'even in these countries deinstitutionalisation eventually came to pass' (ibid., p. 367). Amongst industrialised nations, only in Japan where 'mental illness is still regarded as a great stigma' (ibid., p. 363) did asylums remain a mainstay of the mental health system, and in fact while other nations were closing them down, Japan embarked on an expansion of asylum provision.

There were real economic reasons too for selling them off. They had been expensive to run, staff and maintain, but now that decisions had been made around a great deal of the world to close them, their closure assumed another significance: selling the sites could raise much needed capital to fund the new approach to care within the local community. This was summed up at the time by Korman (1991) as follows:

> The resources tied up in the hospitals are essential for the development of community-based services: capital represented by the buildings and land and revenue as represented by the running costs and expertise of staff.
>
> (p. 12)

We saw in Chapter 1 that many of the large asylums had been built on the outskirts of the big cities: those 'strings of beads' as Clair Wills called the asylums around London. Somewhere in the Treasury it must have become clear that they were sitting on what was becoming more and more valuable real estate land and that the sale of the hospital sites was a means of balancing their precarious budgets (Jones, 1993). The sale price of the Netherne Hospital estate is no longer kept on record, despite a Freedom of Information request made for the purposes of this book, though in 1993 Jones found that 'figures of £40 million–£60 million for the old hospital sites were commonly quoted' (p. 227). These would then have been tidy sums for the then Department of Health, though not it seems to finance a truly effective system of community care. There were clearly 'underlying economic motives' (McCrae and Nolan, p. 166), rather than any meaningful modernisation of mental health care behind the policy of asylum closures. Selling off the asylums and their land, it seemed, 'allowed governments to save money while simultaneous giving their policy a humanitarian gloss' (Scull, 2015, p. 139). In the following decades, there were widespread allegations of asset-stripping: 'funds acquired from the sale of mental hospitals are siphoned into other areas of the health service to the detriment of community mental health care' (Barham, 2020, p. 148), and it wasn't only the real estate on which the old asylums stood which was sold on: 'after the developers moved in, Victorian fireplaces and oak floorboards were sold as architectural salvage' (Taylor, 2014, p. 243)

What replaced the old asylums in many parts of the world was a system which became known in the UK and elsewhere as Care in the Community, and it is important to trace briefly the early development of community care, its impact on former residents of the old psychiatric hospitals and explore what kind of in-patient care remained for those who still needed it.

Community care for the mentally ill had existed for centuries, millennia even, or as McCrae and Nolan (2016) put it: 'In the beginning there was care in the community' (p. 1). In the Middle Ages, monks cared for those in distress out in the community as well as in the monasteries themselves or more usually, families and local communities in one way or another took responsibility for their more vulnerable members. From the 18th century, as we have seen, in the UK, America and many European countries, the responsibility passed to institutions, and 'up to the outbreak of war, the development of mental health services outside the hospitals was patchy and sporadic' (Jones, 1993, p. 141). In the 1940s however, there was 'an emerging trend in the use of psychiatric outpatient clinics by general practitioners' (McCrae & Nolan, 2016, p. 126), and the Netherlands, Norway and Switzerland led the way in social psychiatry (Barham, 2020) in the immediate aftermath of the Second World War. In 1953, the World Health Organization called for a new model for the development of mental health services and a reduction of hospital beds and in 1957 in the UK, the 'Worthing Experiment' aimed to avoid admissions as much as possible with 'most psychiatric referrals receiving outpatient treatment, domiciliary visits or day hospital care' (ibid., p. 157). These early initiatives, in the words of Andrew Solomon (2014), drew on 'a curious mix of valid optimism, economic expediency and ideological rigidity' (p. 312).

Solomon's words could also be applied to a parallel movement which developed in the post-war decades in the field of education: inclusion, or in other words the placing of all children, irrespective of their learning differences or special needs in the same school with the same curriculum (Imray & Colley, 2017). Inclusion shared many of the same hopes, conceptual shifts but also barriers as care in the community. Professor Mike Oliver (1949–2019) was an academic in the field of inclusive education and also was 'an influential critic of residential care' (Jack, 1998), though Johnson and Walmsley (2010) were perhaps the first to draw parallels between the policy shift in education in the UK in the final decades of the 20th century away from 'segregation' in special schools and towards 'inclusion' in mainstream schools, and the closure of the large asylums in favour of 'care in the community.' Johnson and Walmsley showed that the advent of both inclusive education and care in the community were nurtured by the United Nations Universal Declaration of Human Rights (1948) and that the rights discourse also saw both institutionalisation and special schools as an infringement of human rights. This brought about significant conceptual shifts in education in the UK and elsewhere and a 'dogmatic attempt to discontinue special schools' (Allan & Brown, 2001, p. 200), though in education, other than in some countries such as Italy and Australia and a few states in Germany, the wholesale closure of special schools never materialised (Imray & Colley, 2017).

Six years after the United Nations Universal Declaration of Human Rights (1948), the drive towards care in the community for those with mental illness was increasingly underpinned by Government policy and legislation, though it was almost simultaneously dogged by funding and other issues. In the UK in 1954, the Percy Commission had been set up to review legislation with relation to mental illness. Its conclusions, published in 1957, recommended a closer alliance between mental health and general health service and provision and pointed the way towards a more community-centred provision. The Mental

Health Act (1959) enshrined many of the recommendations of the Percy Commission into law and brought a closer alliance with the NHS itself and went some way to creating conditions for effective treatment in the community.

Enoch Powell's 'Water towers' speech of 1961 as we have seen condemned the old 'asylums,' but he did not ignore what could replace them. He said:

> This brings me of course to the complement of the hospital pattern, the pattern of provision in the community. It would be quite unrealistic to attempt to state what is intended, and what is not intended, by way of hospital provision in the 1970s and not to spell out with as much precision and detail as is practicable all that this implies in terms of care outside the hospitals.
> (Powell, 1961)

He was aware though that the 'flow of personnel into community care' would be expensive. If his aim was to be achieved, local authorities would need to be 'armed with the necessary capital provision,' and the endeavour would need to be 'sustained by a widespread public understanding and resolve.' Powell, according to his biographer Simon Heffer in 2008, was becoming increasingly frustrated by these funding issues and by the slow roll-out of care in the community as he had envisaged it.

Although the Seebohm report of 1968 led to the creation by 1970 of an integrated social work profession and in 1973 the first course in Community Psychiatric Nursing was launched at Chiswick College in London (McCrae & Nolan, 2016), successive Labour and Conservative Governments in the UK 'acknowledged, but did not address, the need to provide more resources to deliver mental services in the community' (Turner et al., 2015, p. 602). A reorganisation of the NHS in 1974 had further integrated mental health and general and hospital services under Local Authorities and demanded a new strategy for delivering community-based care. The subsequent Labour government, operating under great financial stringency, accepted the thrust of the reorganisation (Turner et al., 2015) but increased the mental health budget by a mere 1.8%. *Better Services for the Mentally Ill*, published by the Department of Health and Social Security in 1975, promised within 20 years a ninefold increase in accommodation for adults in the community, including private and voluntary-type provision. A National Development group was even set up to oversee and monitor these changes, but it disbanded after five years citing frustration at a lack of policy development and resource allocation (Korman, p. 22).

Throughout the 1970s and 1980s, policies in the UK at least tried to address the gap between the original concept of care in the community and how it was actually playing out, and a subsequent Committee of Enquiry (Cmnd 7648) tried to address the lack of resources by proposing the use of spare housing stock instead of purpose-built community facilities for the mentally ill. The reduction of new purpose-built facilities for people with mental illness and the increased use of council or privately owned housing to accommodate them would continue for the next 40 years.

The oil crisis which began in the early 1970s forced governments to reduce public spending and resourcing still further, and delays in the creation of methods for transferring funds from the old asylums to General Hospitals and to social services further 'undermined community care' (Korman, 1991, p. 27). Korman's (1991) case study of Darenth Park Hospital in Kent as the local service transitioned from the closure of the hospital to care in the community is stark in its predictions of issues which would bedevil care in the community almost from its inception:

> Local authorities might feel no incentive to provide funds for people they see as the responsibility of the health service, especially if clients coming out of hospital are in competition with residents of the local community for the use of limited resources. Hospital residents may do worse under this arrangement than they did before and community care would continue to be somewhat chaotic representing poor value for money, providing an inadequate range of services for some, and none to others. . . . Discharge into the community might make people with mental health conditions worse.
>
> (p. 54)

It was gradually becoming clear then that 'changing the pattern of provision within the NHS would prove easier than persuading social services to provide for highly dependent people who had spent most of their lives in the mental institutions' (McCrae & Nolan, p. 163), and as 'the wrecking balls swung through the old asylums, it became evident that care in the community could be good, or cheap, but not both' (Jay, p. 193).

In other countries, policies to promote care in the community instead of in large institutions followed a similar pattern of hope, followed by disappointment. In the United States in 1961, the National Institute for Mental Health issued a report, *Action for Mental Health* and in 1963, John F. Kennedy launched a major federal investment in community mental health centres (McCrae & Nolan, 2016). There were some successful experiments in the use of community facilities to support people with mental illness, such as the ENCOR programme in eastern Nebraska, but federal community mental health services were based almost solely on a medical model and largely ignored the basic needs of accommodation, meals, clothing and income (Korman, 1991). Welfare payments increasingly funded the growth of private nursing homes and care homes in which large numbers were confined. In an echo of the private madhouses which had sprung up in the 18th and 19th centuries, this became 'an entrepreneurial industry, which profited from human misery' (Scull, p. 376.), with these facilities often staffed by former employees of the old asylums. Like in the UK, houses run by voluntary associations, private providers or housing associations as well as bed and breakfasts proliferated in the 1990s, and 'opening a home for people leaving a psychiatric hospital was a potentially lucrative venture' (McCrae & Nolan, 2016, p. 275). Care in the community was turning into 'a shell game with no pea' (ibid., p. 369) – a con trick with no substance.

In Italy, where asylums had been closed so rapidly, alternative structures had not been provided fast enough. The academic and social historian Kathleen Jones (1922–2010) undertook two study tours of Italy in the 1980s and disclosed the failure of the community care programme 'with homelessness of ex-patients (known as the *abbandonati)*, inadequate community resources, and poorly funded residual backwards in the old hospitals still in use' (Jack, 1998). The burden in Italy and elsewhere fell to families or former patients were placed in private residential facilities. Australia developed a substantial private medical sector, though funded publicly through the Health Insurance Commission as well as through private health insurance schemes (Rosen, 2006), and although from the early 1970s some community health teams were put in place nationally, they were often idealistically focused on primary prevention, and offered mainly generic services within office hours only. In France, although there was 'a new paradigm in psychiatric care, with a shift from large residential institutions to community-based services' (Coldefy & Curtis, 2010, p. 2125), the original regional asylums were often retained or converted to a more community-focused model.

So, what were the lived experiences of those former asylum residents who found themselves caught up in what Solomon (2014) referred to as 'this social experiment called *deinstitutionalisation*' (p. 312)? A BBC TV *Brass Tacks* documentary in 1982 called 'Doing the Rounds' highlighted the plight of a drifting population of former patients the community was struggling to support. The mentally ill were still with us, it reported, but were now very much left to fend for themselves. In 2010, another BBC documentary *A History of the Madhouse* interviewed former patients who had been discharged in the first years of the care in community initiative. There were those who initially had felt positive about the move, with one using the term 'emancipation' and another saying, 'the best thing was being free.' Another found 'a new self-confidence,' while others remembered the growth of the patient advocacy or 'user movement' around that time, saying 'we could set goals for ourselves.' Taylor (2014) also acknowledged that 'here in a home for "vulnerable adults," I had my first glimpse of adult independence' (p. 191).

This was though, the documentary went on, a honeymoon period for care in the community. The asylums had closed but this hadn't changed the 'often-troubled lives they left behind.' Nor was it always easy for the nursing staff to adapt to the new ways of caring in the community. Many simply 'took their former institutional practices and attitudes from one setting and transferred the same ways of working into the new' (Hardcastle et al., 2007, p. 17). Some of the newer staff in these settings were also frequently not trained nurses and 'resorted to a controlling regime' (McCrae & Nolan, 2016, p. 276)

In July 1990, the Labour MP for Islington North, Jeremy Corbyn, described a state of 'panic' among patients at Friern Hospital, and demanded assurances that the hospital's closure would not proceed unless adequate accommodation for its inmates could be guaranteed (Taylor, 2014, p. 117). His fears were well founded: one of the former patients interviewed in the BBC documentary, although initially enthusiastic about her move out into the community, found herself living in a house with 'no bulbs, no carpet and nothing to cook on.' Nor was the reception she and others like her received in the community as warm and welcoming as both Enoch Powell MP and George Gardner MP had hoped for. The community was getting cold feet, old prejudices resurfaced and more than one of the people interviewed felt still ignored and stigmatised. As Andrew Solomon put it in his book *The Noonday Demon: An Anatomy of Depression:*

> The truly depressed were not made invisible by asylums; they had always been largely invisible because their very disease causes them to sever human contacts.
>
> (p. 318)

All over the world, 'the burden that the hospitals had been carrying was more than the community could bear' (Jay, 2016, p. 193). This certainly was the case in the United States where insurance companies pared back on provision for mental illness and former patients ended up in grim hostels or on the street (ibid.) and were soon labelled 'sidewalk psychotics' (Scull, 2015, p. 376).

Care in the community, it seemed, was fast becoming at best 'a kind of shared myth' without clear definition (Turner et al., 2015) and at worst a 'synonym for neglect' (Jay, 2016, p. 225). Barbara Taylor in *The Last Asylum* (2014) highlighted two unintended ways that cost was being mitigated. In an interview with service user activist Peter Campbell, Taylor quotes him as saying: 'Community Care is built on medication' (Taylor, 2014, p. 258). In other words, if there was once a problem with relatively unaccountable overuse of medication in the hospitals to keep patients compliant, that was still an issue out in the community. Taylor also points to the role of women in providing for free, what was supposed to have been provided by the state: 'When politicians talk about "community care," what they really mean is women: women inside and outside families; women struggling often with meagre resources to look after their loved ones' (p. 82). Janet Finch and other feminist writers had warned of this 30 years earlier when arguing for the retention of residential care 'as a means of promoting the right of women to avoid the oppression of the caring role enforced on them' (Jack, 1998, p. 24).

There were a number of campaigns, political statements and initiatives over the last decades of the 20th century, though many were concerned with the perceived shortcomings of care in the community rather than the process and practice of in-patient care itself. For example, in 1988, *Community Care – Agenda for Action*, otherwise known as 'The Griffiths Report,' was published following an audit commission warning about the difficulties of delivering care in the community. The report stated baldly that community care remained 'a poor relation: everybody's distant relative, but nobody's baby' (p. iv). The report further reinforced the role of 'managerialism' within the NHS and also promoted the use of the private sector in mental health care, an issue which continues to be debated today, with Hudson (2021) finding that 'the post-1980 period can be characterised as one in which the inherently paternalistic nature of this (professional – client) relationship was challenged by "consumerism," a model thought to be better equipped for meeting individual needs and preferences' (p. 5).

As criticisms of the way care in the community had been enacted started to ramp up, the speed of closure of the old institutions also came under fire across the political divide. In 1996, UK Conservative Prime Minister John Major wrote a letter to the Secretary of State for Health (Jack, 1998) expressing serious concern over the policy of community care for mentally ill people and suggested that 'the programme of closure of the mental hospitals may have gone too far' (ibid., p. 8). Just a year later, Frank Dobson, the Secretary of State for Labour in the New Labour Government, had declared in the House of Commons that 'Care in the Community has failed.'

Concerns around the safety of the mentally ill and of those around them continued to dominate debates and 'since the 1990s there has come about a drastic change of attitude as to what constitutes an acceptable risk in mental health care' (Barham, 2020, p. 19). In 1993, a new white paper *Health of the Nation*, delivered by the Department of Health, placed a 'heavy emphasis on the prevention of suicide' (Jones, p. 234) with two of the three primary targets for mental health outlined in the document being directly concerned with reducing suicide numbers. Whilst targets such as these can hardly be argued against, Jones (1993) suggests that they might have been actually a 'reflection of the need to find something measurable in a field unamenable to medical statistics, rather than an attempt to address the real issues of social care' (p. 235).

What was created for the seriously ill were much smaller in-patient psychiatric units in or very near to general hospitals, though these settings were essentially clinical rather than residential (McRae & Nolan, p. 200), and very much resembled the wards in a general hospital. This model of small in-patient units, usually offering about 30 beds per unit, is essentially what exists today. In 2004, the Sainsbury Centre for Mental Health (SCMH) – a charity which works to improve the quality of life for people with severe mental health problems – in association with the National Institute for Mental Health in England undertook a national survey of in-patient wards in England. Some of their key findings would still resonate 20 years later: almost a quarter of ward managers reported that their wards did not serve their purpose, only just over half the wards surveyed had sufficient quiet areas for service users and less than half had appropriate areas for service users to meet with friends and relatives, and despite a clear evidence base, psychosocial interventions were not routinely available on most in-patient wards.

One thing however remained more or less unchanged: the Mental Health Act 1983, though like many Acts of Parliament, it had been amended over time and principally by the Mental Health (Amendment) Act of 2007. The Government's original intention at that time (Lawton-Smith, 2008) had been to pass a wholly new Mental Health Act to replace the Act of 1983 in response to renewed concerns about risks to the public posed by people with a serious mental disorder living in the community. However, following 'a long-fought battle' (Turner et al., 2015, p. 603) between the Government and an alliance of bodies seeking to improve mental health care more generally, only amendments, rather than the wholesale replacement of the 1983 legislation, were passed. These 2007 amendments reinforce the conditions for legal confinement both in hospital and in the community and also extend the powers of those able to apply compulsory detention orders to a larger range of medical practitioners, replacing 'approved social workers' with the broader 'approved mental health professionals.' Objections to these 2007 amendments were centred on concerns that people's dignity, autonomy and human rights had been overlooked, and campaigns continue today for a comprehensive reform of mental health legislation.

Of particular relevance to my own lived experience of in-patient care in 2020 was *The Five Year Forward View for Mental Health* drawn up by the independent Mental Health Taskforce (2016), which brought together in 2015 leaders in mental health care, service users and other stakeholders. Its report was published in February 2016 for implementation by 2020–2021. There is an acknowledgement at the beginning of the 82-page report of a 'need to re-energise and improve mental health care across the NHS to meet increased demand and improve outcomes' (p. 5) and that a 'fresh mindset' would be needed. Despite the 39% reduction of adult in-patient psychiatric beds in the years between 1998 and 2012, the 'severity of need and the number of people being detained under the Mental Health Act continues to increase, suggesting opportunities to intervene earlier are being missed' (p. 9). Bed occupancy had risen for the fourth consecutive year prior to the report and 'pressure on beds had been exacerbated by a lack of early intervention and crisis care' (p. 9), with the resulting shortage leading to 'people being transferred long distances outside of their area' (p. 9). Alarmingly, it found that many acute wards are 'not always safe, therapeutic or conducive to recovery' (p. 9). There was a further concern that 'men of African and Caribbean heritage are up to 6.6 times more likely to be admitted as inpatients or detained under the Mental Health Act, indicating a systemic failure to provide effective crisis care for these groups' (p. 9).

As it should, the report gives a great deal of attention to suicide prevention. and this has also been the subject of policy documents such as the 2002

Department of Health National Suicide Prevention Strategy for England, and the 2019 Cross Government Suicide Prevention Workplan, but of the Taskforce's 58 recommendations which needed to be enacted by the year 2020/2021, only 6 reference in-patient care directly only 6 directly concern in-patient care, and arguably only the last 4 are specifically about the nature and practice of in-patient care itself:

- Recommendation 15: 'By 2020/21, NHS England should support at least 30,000 more women each year to access evidence-based specialist mental health care during the perinatal period. This should include access to . . . the right range of specialist community or inpatient care' (p. 33).
- Recommendation 18: 'By 2020/21, NHS England should invest to ensure that no acute hospital is without all-age mental health liaison services in emergency departments and inpatient wards' (p. 34).
- Recommendation 20: 'NHS England and PHE (Public Health England) should support all mental health inpatient units . . . to be smoke-free by 2018' (p. 34).
- Recommendation 22: 'The practice of sending people out of area for acute inpatient care as a result of local acute bed pressures is eliminated entirely by no later than 2020/21' (p. 35).
- Recommendation 31: 'NHS England should work with CCGs (Clinical Commissioning Groups), local authorities and other partners to develop and trial a new model of acute inpatient care for young adults aged 16–25' (p. 40).
- Recommendation 56: 'The Department of Health should ensure that the scope of the Healthcare Safety Investigation Branch includes deaths from all causes in inpatient mental health settings' (p. 63).

In 1993, Jones had found that 'in the medical enthusiasm for the district general hospital model, arguments that psychiatric patients needed a different kind of architecture and use of space from general hospital patients because they were ambulant and needed occupation and social activities, were ignored' (p. 182). Despite this warning, there are only three references in the *Five Year Forward Plan* to the 'environment' of in-patient care and only one mentions the importance of an environment that 'maximises opportunities for rehabilitation,' though there is no detail in the report of what these environments should look like or of the nature of therapeutic care which should be carried on within them.

It was in just such an environment I found myself more than 35 years after being discharged from Netherne Hospital. My illness from 1985 had returned. It had a new more detailed clinical name: 'severe agitated depression with psychotic features,' but it presented in very similar ways to the 'nervous disorder' recorded in my notes in Netherne Hospital. I knew of course that mental health care had changed in that time, but naively I underestimated exactly how much . . .

References

Allan, J., & Brown, S. (2001). Special Schools and Inclusion. *Educational Review*, 53(2), 199–207.

Barham, P. (2020). *Closing the Asylum – The Mental Patient in Modern Society*. London: Process Press.

BBC. (1982). Doing the Rounds. *BBC Brass Tacks*. June 24th 1982.

BBC/Open University. (2010). *A History of the Madhouse* (First broadcast May 17th, 2010). London: BBC.

Coldefy, M., & Curtis, S. (2010). The Geography of Institutional Psychiatric Care in France 1800–2000: Historical Analysis of the Spatial Diffusion of Specialised Facilities for Institutional Care of Mental Illness. *Social Science & Medicine*, 71(2010), 2117–2129.

Department of Health and Social Security. (1975). *Better Services for the Mentally Ill*. (Cmnd 6233). London: HMSO.

Disused Burial Grounds Act. (1884). London: HMSO. www.legislation.gov.uk/ukpga/ Vict/47-48/72/contents (accessed August 26th 2023).

Dobson, F. (1997). *Frank Dobson Outlines Third Way for Mental Health Services* (press release). HMSO: Department of Health.

Griffiths, R. (1988). *Community Care Agenda for Action: A Report to the Secretary of State for Social Services*. London: HMSO.

Gumb, J. (1994). Last Few Patients Leave Netherne. *The Mirror*. August 11th 1994.

Hardcastle, M., Kennard, D., Grandison, S., & Fagin L. (Eds.). (2007). *Experiences of Mental Health In-patient Care Narratives from Service Users, Carers and Professionals*. Hove: Routledge.

Heffer, S. (2008). *Like the Roman: The Life of Enoch Powell*. London: Faber and Faber.

Hudson, B. (2021). *Clients, Consumers or Citizens? The Privatisation of Adult Social Care in England*. Bristol: Bristol University Press.

Imray, P., & Colley, A. (2017). *Inclusion is Dead: Long Live Inclusion*. London: Routledge.

Jack, R. (Ed.). (1998). *Residential Versus Community Care: The Role of Institutions in Welfare Provision*. London: Macmillan Press Ltd.

Jay, M. (2016). *This Way Madness Lies*. London: Thames and Hudson.

Johnson, K., Walmsley, J., with Wolfe, M. (2010). *People with Intellectual Disabilities – Towards a Good Life?* Bristol: The Policy Press.

Jones, K. (1993). *Asylums and After: A Revised History of the Mental Health Services: From the Early 18th Century to the 1990's*. London: Athlone.

Kings Fund. (2015). *Making Change Possible: Case study 1: Deinstitutionalisation in UK Mental Health Services*. The King's Fund. www.kingsfund.org.uk.

Korman, N. (1991). *Managing Change: The Development of Mental Handicap Services in Southeast Thames Regional Health Authority, 1978–88*, PhD thesis. London School of Economics and Political Science.

Lawton-Smith, S. (2008). *The Mental Health Act 2007: Ideas that Change Health Care*. The King's Fund. www.kingsfund.org.uk.

Mental Health Taskforce. (2016). *Five Year Forward Plan for Mental Health: A Report from the Independent Mental Health Taskforce to the NHS in England*. www.england.nhs.uk/mentalhealth/taskforce (accessed August 28th 2023).

McCrae, N., & Nolan, P. (2016). *The Story of Nursing in British Mental Hospitals: Echoes from the Corridors*. Abingdon: Routledge.

Powell, E. (1961). Address to the National Association for Mental Health. In *Emerging Patterns for the Mental Health Services and the Public*. London: NAMH.

Rosen, A. (2006). Australia's National Mental Health Strategy in Historical Perspective: Beyond the Frontier. *Bulletin of the Board of International Affairs of the Royal College of Psychiatrists*, 3(3).

Sainsbury Centre for Mental Health (SCMH). (2004). *A National Survey of Psychiatric Wards in England*. London: SCMH Publications.

SAVE. (1995). *Mind over Matter: A Study of the Country's Threatened Mental Asylums*. London: SAVE Britain's Heritage.

Scull, A. (2015). *Madness in Civilization: A Cultural History of Insanity from the Bible to Freud, from the Madhouse to Modern Medicine*. London: Thames and Hudson.

Solomon, A. (2014). *The Noonday Demon: An Anatomy of Depression*. London: Vintage Books.

Taylor, B. (2014). *The Last Asylum*. London: Penguin.

The Seebohm Report. (1968). *Journal of the Institute of Health Education*, 6(3), 22–33 (Cmnd 3703). https://doi.org/10.1080/03073289.1968.10799793

Turner J., Hayward, R., Angel, K., Fulford, B., Hall, J., Millard C., & Thomson, M. (2015). The History of Mental Health Services in Modern England: Practitioner Memories and the Direction of Future Research. *Medical History*, 59(4), 599–624.

5 In-patient provision in the 21st century

A ward in a house at a provision within a service, near a hospital

The policy landscape of in-patient mental health care in the autumn of 2020 had been formed by legislation dating back at least 40 years, by formal and informal guidance, by opinion, counter-opinion and concerns for the safety of service users and those around them. It had also been formed by a desire never to return to what were perceived to be the bad old days of the asylums.

My experience of this new landscape would be in line with every region of England and the devolved nations: it was in a ward in a facility built about 20 years before to replace a large Victorian asylum which had previously been a workhouse. This new facility had been given a name rich in English heritage followed by the word 'unit,' but this was fairly quickly changed to 'house.' It was part of a provision, within a service, near a General Hospital and was administered by an NHS Trust, though confusingly not the same Trust as the General Hospital on whose grounds it stood. And I was a 'service user.'

I will try to describe my own lived experience of that ward in the autumn of 2020. This will not be, unless absolutely necessary, an account of my own deteriorating state of mind, but rather the environment, resources, people and activity of the ward itself. The description is structured similarly to my account in Chapter 3 of Netherne Hospital in the autumn of 1985. It is not fair though to draw exact comparisons between these two very different settings, separated by nearly four decades and a bewildering tapestry of political and social changes. I do so simply to lay the groundwork for a debate which will be carried on in Chapter 7 when we ask what has been gained and what has been lost since the closing of the large asylums.

This part of the book has been very difficult to write. I said at the end of Chapter 3 that my experience in Netherne Hospital in 1985 was generally speaking positive, but I cannot say the same of the similar length of time I spent on a ward 35 years later. I accept in this and other chapters based around my own lived experience that 'psychiatric in-patient wards look very different depending on your position in relation to them' (Hardcastle et al., 2007, p. xxi). I was very ill when I was admitted to the ward, and my condition worsened significantly during the 12 weeks I spent there. My memory of those months and my emotions must at the very least be coloured by my

DOI: 10.4324/9781003455042-5

mental state of the time. I was also admitted while the coronavirus pandemic was still at its height, and this inevitably affected the services and atmosphere on the ward in seen and unseen ways. For these reasons, I am grateful to service users Amy and Caroline who spent time in the same provision between 2018 and 2020. They agreed to share some of their experiences, which I have included here alongside my own to provide an alternative voice and examples of lived experience before the restrictions of the Covid-19 pandemic.

The trauma of those months is still very real: I have flashbacks of my time on that ward, but I have no anger towards the clinical and other staff in the way I did for many years towards the consultant psychiatrist described in Chapter 2. It is also important to say that work continues to be done since 2020 to improve the environments on this and other wards, though I have not been back to check.

In the month or so before my admission, I was supported in various ways in the community: by my excellent GP, by the community team, by the Integrated Delivery Team and by the crisis teams. Despite the coronavirus pandemic, I was visited in person by some kind, and hugely supportive people, people who for reasons I was yet to understand, really didn't want me to have to go into hospital: *It's not the right environment*; *we need to keep you out of there*, or more darkly: *it's not in a good place right now*.

Phone contact was less effective, although on one morning I spoke to a nurse whose gentle Scottish lilt and kind words reduced me to floods of tears. On another occasion though when I phoned the crisis team, the person on the other end of the line listened to my woes and said this:

It sounds like you need some more dopamine.

This was the medical model of mental health care writ large and applied by someone who I like to think was maybe at the end of a long shift trying to say the right thing to people like me. But it is also a deficit model: mental illness as a lack of something. I had heard this more than 50 years before when as a young boy I had said to what was then known as the 'family doctor,' that I felt 'funny.' I don't remember the context, and the language of mental illness was certainly not part of my vocabulary at the time, but this was the first time I had tried to articulate my complicated feelings. That GP was highly regarded locally, and with good reason: barely 20 years before he had been a prisoner of war in Japan, had suffered unimaginable hardships and somehow survived. He said:

What you need is some steel in your spine.

And that was that.

But neither steel nor more dopamine in 2020 helped, and so I took the now common route to a mental health in-patient ward: via the Accident and

Emergency (A&E) Department of the local General Hospital. I was lucky though: I only spent a few hours on A&E on a bed tucked into a corner somewhere. I subsequently met people who had spent a lot longer than me alongside the broken legs, the heart attacks and the other conditions which bring people to Emergency Departments, waiting for a bed to become free for them on a mental health ward, hopefully near to home, though all too often hundreds of miles away: a young woman for example – maybe 19 or 20 – charming, bright, personable but in the midst of some terrible crisis – spent two weeks in A&E before a bed was found for her on my ward.

In the autumn of 2020, Healthwatch,[1] an organisation funded by the UK Department for Health and Social Care, was drawing up what is called *The 15 step challenge*, which aimed to improve the first impressions service users have on entering a ward. In my case it took a lot more than 15 steps to reach the in-patient ward, but nevertheless, these are my own first impressions: following a meeting with some very attentive people from another 'team,' I was accompanied over the road, up the loading bay and through the double doors of the modern building which would be my home for the next 12 weeks. Then, through a first set of security doors, along one corridor, turn left, through another set of security doors, along another corridor; through a third set of security doors into what felt like some kind of liminal space between two worlds; behind us the semi-normal world of offices and meeting rooms, and there, behind another set of heavy doors and reinforced windows: the ward itself. Those doors are pushed open, and I am inside. Amy describes this experience as *surreal*, and it is the right word: the stuff of dreams, where time is fluid and reality becomes distorted.

Immediately opposite the entrance: the nurses' station behind large windows – phones, computer screens, boxes, files, bags, coats, crisp packets, people talking, reading files, looking at lists on the wall. The beating heart of an acute ward but also, I would learn, the target of violence and abuse, the wooden door smashed more than once in the next few weeks. The ward itself: a long corridor. This is what surprised me the most. These were the stuff of the old asylums, weren't they? The bad old days. A third of a mile in a straight line at Rainhill Hospital near Liverpool (Jones, 1993), nearly as far in a curve at Netherne. Often ranked alongside the water towers and the chimneys as symbols of all the impersonal machinery of the institutions, and yet here we were again: a long corridor stretching either side of the nurses' station: female one end, male the other, with bedrooms on either side, 20 in all, and other rooms: storerooms, activity rooms. All locked. Sterile, neutral colours, and clean, hard edges. Some display boards in reinforced cabinets. A few dark blue chairs: slightly more comfortable than in an office but much less comfortable than at home. Not many chairs actually . . . they didn't tend to last long. And low ceilings, with those lights which are meant to replicate 'natural' light, because actually, along this long corridor there was no natural light other than from windows in the rooms along its edge. But there would be no darkness either I would learn. The lights always on so no one was ever out of sight.

For Amy, it was her first mental hospital admission, and as well as the *fear, shame and self-stigma* she described, she was shocked by the fact that so many of the normal things of daily life were taken away from her:

> *Just because someone has a serious mental health condition and needs residential psychiatric help, doesn't mean their basic needs can be ignored, but there was the inability to wear necklaces, and the lack of access to electric cables for mobile or gadget charging. One night staff could not locate my hairdryer and I had to try to sleep with wet hair, which was awful and defeated the point of my ward admission which was for rest. I was lucky to have access to my own mobile phone. Some patients were not even able to bring in a change of clothes.*

My own bedroom: this is the place which still haunts me. I wake up sometimes in the night and I think I am still there. Panicked, I wake my wife to reassure me that I am not. Not just the bedroom itself: the terrible things that happened there, but it is the bedroom itself I will try to capture here. And because this whole building contrived to deny us natural light and at least a glimpse of the outside world whenever it could, I will start with the window.

In 1900, Ernest White, medical superintendent of the City of London Mental Hospital in Dartford, wrote: 'the more glass you have in an asylum the less you have broken' (McCrae & Nolan, 2016, p. 48). This was not a therapeutic message which had survived over the next 120 years. The window was small: about a metre square with thick reinforced glass, and a thick dark brown metal frame. It was of the heavy 'slider' type so that you could open only half of it, but not so it was then 'open,' because the opening itself was covered in a metal mesh screen. Air could get in, but not much light. Secret smokers on the ward would sit with their faces right up against this mesh and blow their smoke out through it.

The view from this window, potentially, was nice: green, the edge of parkland, trees, rabbits, but these were all filtered through the dark brown mesh and reinforced glass. One bright, frosty late autumn morning, a care assistant who I came to know and like immensely came into my room. My flimsy blue curtains were still closed. He drew them back and pointed through the glass. *Look at that, Andrew*, he said, *can't you see how beautiful that is?* I couldn't.

There was another window. A small internal one in the door designed so that you could be observed at all times, and in the top corner of the ceiling opposite the door, a multi-angle mirror so that no one could hide. Everyone was on suicide watch all the time, and it was through this small window that throughout the night, every 30 minutes – or 15 minutes if you had been judged of higher risk – one of the care staff would shine a torch. *Just to check you are still with us, Andrew* commented a nurse with dark humour. It was an indignity and an inconvenience which was easy to justify: there had been many suicides on this ward – almost certainly in this very room – and on wards all over the country. Caroline remembers the all too regular intrusions of the torch and other night-time disruptions:

> *Sleeping was hard. Staff shone a torch through the door at you every half an hour. There was often lots of noise when patients were brought in in the middle of the night and they were swearing and kicking things. Quite scary to listen to. I had a girl in the room next to me who insisted on playing rap music with swear words in it 24/7. It was horrendous and made me really upset. It was only after asking for days that I finally got moved to another room!*

I am keen to move on now from my room in that ward as it triggers memories I would rather not have and images I would really rather not see, so I am going to keep it short. An 'en-suite,' but only in name: an alcove with a simple shower, toilet with no seat or lid and a sink all operated with push buttons – the whole separated from the room itself by a flimsy screen. Mine fell down and was never replaced so that lying in bed I was a few feet away from the toilet. The shower had a short curtain but mine was removed for my own safety. Amy remembers the shower like this:

> *The shower in my room did not run hot, it reached lukewarm at best and this intermittency was apparently a common problem. This was problematic for me with long hair when I needed a hair wash.*

On the female end of the long corridor, Amy recalls, there was a shared bathroom but as everywhere else on the ward, patient safety was prioritised and there was little privacy:

> *At that time patients could bathe by themselves, which helped me to relax, but by the time of my departure staff were required to accompany patients. However, again I assume because of the potential weapon risk they posed, sanitary bins were not provided in the shared bathroom area. This meant when it was time for my period, I transported any of my used products along the corridor to my bedroom bin as discreetly as possible. I mentioned this to the ward matron before I left as I did not want others to suffer the same embarrassment.*

Each bedroom had a solid desk built into the wall and a hard round foam seat with no back. Amy describes this seat as a 'pouffe,' which is accurate, except it could not in any way be described as soft or comfortable. This was particularly difficult for Amy, as old injuries meant she could not sit comfortably without lumbar support, a condition made worse when she was stressed:

> I explained to the staff that I could not support myself seated and that I had no comfortable way to sit in my room. One member of staff took me on a tour so I could point out a chair that could give me respite, however the use of an office chair was declined. I now understand that this was because some patients may use a hard chair as a weapon, but it left me in considerable pain. No one asked if I would like paracetamol to assist this.

There was also a built-in cupboard with no door and no clothes rail – and the bed. This was at once a place of torture and of refuge and was not designed for comfort: narrow and too short for me, the mattress was hard and covered with a shiny synthetic material in that same dark blue, with sheets so small and thin that they would not stay on the bed. At the worst of my illness, I would spend so many hours in this bed with a sheet over my head, often from straight after supper at 5:30 p.m. till 8 a.m. the next morning, that I began to develop sores on my legs and back. Bed sores – in 2020 – on a mental health ward. That doesn't sound right.

The term 'ligature point' is very much part of the lexicon of modern mental health care today. It means anything from which it might be possible to fix a rope, or wire, or cable. I won't spell out the reasons why. Any normal house or flat is covered in potential ligature points, except they are not called that. They are the pictures on the walls, the wardrobes, the shelves, the taps, the coat hooks, the bed posts, the stairs, the doors, the light fittings. I could go on. Everything which makes a place a home: personal or functional. My room, like everywhere else on the ward, had had all potential ligature points removed. As James Mumford notes in his 2022 article 'Therapy Beyond Good and Evil' in *The New Atlantic* about his own in-patient experience: 'How many ways of suicide have been attempted here? They must have worked most of them out by now' (p. 29). The environment of the modern-day mental health ward has been reduced to a series of bland, flat and unadorned surfaces, but at what cost to the well-being of the people who have to stay there? Let's leave my room behind now though. Please.

There were two rooms not routinely locked: the television room and the dining room. The television room had a large TV screen on the wall in a secure and locked glass-fronted unit. So, theoretically, residents could watch television whenever they wanted, except there were only one or two chairs, and the remote control had been lost, as had the key to the unit, so it was not possible to change channels. I didn't know before I went into that ward that there was such a thing as *Forces TV*, but I do now because that was the channel the TV was permanently tuned to, presumably at the request of one of the many service veterans who spent time on the ward.

Medication was distributed at a small hatch beside the nurses' room. With more available medications than 40 years before, the chart listing your drugs got longer or shorter as the clinical team tried to find the combination which would mean you could, possibly, go home. Amy was left feeling that in this there was *a real disconnect between mental and physical medical treatments:*

> *At no point did any of the staff ask what other medication I took or if there was a need to continue with the contraceptive pill to regulate my hormones. At one point I rang my GP and asked them to relay my existing conditions and medicine, which they did. But I think my ability to communicate that requirement was unusual.*

Most of the available chairs ended up in the dining room, though here again, as Caroline recalls:

> *Mealtimes were hard. Some patients were unpredictable and would shout and throw things.*

Lunch and dinner had to be ordered the day before and if you didn't manage to do that, you just got a sandwich of someone else's choosing. I don't remember much about the food. It certainly wasn't bad, but I do remember tapioca once again, which was strangely reassuring. What was slightly unusual were the times of meals: lunch at 12 and dinner at 5:30 with the addition of a bedtime serving of toast and milk. A kind of return to childhood. Frustratingly, there was no consistent way of getting a cup of tea or coffee during the day and the small kitchen was locked. You could ask a member of staff to make you one and they often obliged, but they usually had far more pressing things to do – like trying to stop people killing themselves. Periodically, a trolley with tea, coffee, milk, sometimes biscuits and a flask of not too hot water was wheeled out, but it was often overturned, and, like the chairs, mugs were few and far between. As soon as I had recovered in January 2021, I sent the ward a box of plastic mugs. It was the least I could do.

There was also the activity room, with posters on the walls, books, DVD's, board games and jigsaws, and big blue bean bags to sink into. A nice environment and one which did not follow the normal pattern of bland ligature-free conformity. This was almost certainly why it was also locked and only accessible when at least two staff were present. We went there quite a lot though, especially in the evenings, but on several occasions it was out of use because staff meetings were being held in it, or through the window you could glimpse one member of staff in tears and being comforted by another usually older and more senior nurse. I think the consultants had their own room to cry in.

There was also a laundry room, locked obviously and not accessible other than with a member of staff. The idea behind this room was a good one: two washing machines and a dryer available free of charge for service users to allow them to take responsibility for their own laundry. Maintain a bit of independence. Except, firstly, this room served two wards, or about 40 people, and one of the machines was broken down from the day I arrived to the day I left – that's about 12 weeks. There were service users, and I was one of them, who were lucky enough to have family and friends who were prepared to take their washing home with them, but many did not have such loved ones. I found out about two years after leaving the ward that there was still only one working washing machine. That's a lot of washing not done, a lot of vulnerable people wearing the same dirty clothes day after day. So, let's quickly go outside, because it will also allow me to talk, and not for the first or last time in this book, about smoking.

The 'courtyard' – and again please bear in mind here that my perceptions were blunted by illness, and that outdoor areas in mental health wards are constantly under review – but I think this was without doubt the most bleak and depressing outdoor recreation space anywhere I have come across. Ever. Caroline agreed:

> *The courtyard was horrible. It was used all day by smokers and there were cigarette butts dropped everywhere. I never set foot in there. It was depressing because I was desperate for some fresh air, and it was a while before I was well enough to go by myself for a walk on the heath.*

There was some grass, but also weeds and concrete and some outdoor furniture, but this was not from a garden centre, light and colourful. These chairs were solid and filled with sand, possibly even concrete. You could not move, let alone throw them. The courtyard was surrounded on three sides by other buildings with windows looking out from offices, wards, corridors. The fourth side was an enormous wooden fence, maybe 20 feet high, though someone did once make it to the top, helped by others and by a stack of furniture, and there they sat, for hours. The fear that they would jump was palpable. A young male nurse, maybe 19 or 20 and possibly not even fully qualified, talked them down. That's a skill not many boys of that age possess. So what was this outdoor space for? Exercise: yes, and some people did walk up and down. Fresh air: certainly, and sunlight: in short supply even out there behind the walls and the giant fence. Principally though it was for smoking.

Recommendation 20 in *The Five Year Forward View for Mental Health* that all mental health in-patient units should be smoke-free by 2018 had not come to pass. At least not on this ward, and I suspect many others across the country. Shortly after my arrival, a date was set when the whole unit – inside and out – would finally be smoke-free, so two years late, but at last it was going to happen. Notices were put up to inform people of the new policy. *That'll last about 5 minutes*, said the man standing next to me. He was right. Shortly after the lights came on that morning and people began emerging from their rooms, the door to the courtyard – which had been locked for the night – was kicked in and the many smokers on the ward simply walked out and lit up. From then on, the courtyard was the smoking area. Access was controlled by a timetable, which meant access to exercise, fresh air and sunlight was restricted for all, especially non-smokers. Amy though recalls that, in a time just before the coronavirus pandemic in the same provision, there were opportunities to get some fresh air other than in the bleak courtyard:

> *If well enough, there were spaces on excursions accompanied by staff a couple of times a week, with spaces limited. This went into the local town centre or a local parkland where on one occasion I was lucky enough to be one of three patients able to walk two therapy dogs for an hour. I remember my joy being out of hospital in nature, seeing blackberries, dragonflies and giant pinecones on the ground and having an affinity with the Labrador I was guiding on a lead . . . I once was able to garden in an internal courtyard garden alongside the gym, weeding and planting pansies bought by an occupational therapist. This was my happiest afternoon during my stay in hospital as it brought an element of normality as gardening is a passion of mine.*

So, what did we do all day? There were activities on offer certainly, though they were sometimes delayed or cancelled: art, though not art therapy, music, games, chess, relaxation, mindfulness for some, anxiety management for others, ward rounds, one-to-one chats with staff. Amy and Caroline, who were in hospital shortly before Covid, remember a richer programme of activities on the ward:

> *Group nail varnishing sessions, baking, singing and once during my stay, art therapy. Every night there was group meditation sessions if wanted, and games or a film. I went to the hospital gym every time I was offered it. I think this was about 5 mornings a week because it made me feel better. I did yoga or used a running machine or sometimes just used the time to go into the smaller sunny courtyard garden outside which was quiet.*
>
> *I went to creative writing and the material just flowed. I wrote poems and pieces of descriptive writing, one of which was framed and put up on the wall in the ward. . . . Other things I enjoyed were table tennis in the gym, walks on the heath, dog walking, nail painting, mindfulness, dominoes, arts and crafts activities, colouring and photography.*

There were no jobs, paid or otherwise, to keep the patients occupied, as there had been in Netherne decades before and in mental hospitals the world over for centuries. One adorable lady, who sang nursery rhymes all day – which sounds annoying but for some reason wasn't – decided to give herself a little job: *just to help out* as she said. She was going to make it her job to sweep up all the cigarette butts in the courtyard and told me she had asked for a broom so that she could get on with it. I said I'd help. We sat there in silence for a while. *When did you ask for the broom,* I asked. *About three weeks ago,* she replied.

Meaningful contact with family and friends was problematic. Caroline describes her concerns:

> *I missed my family terribly and worried about my young children and how my illness would affect them.*

At the time of her admission, Amy's daughter was also very young, and she missed her terribly:

> *The worst thing about being in hospital is being away from your loved ones – human or pet – as much as your own home. The lack of good signal or WiFi connection made it incredibly hard to talk privately to my young daughter. There was shared use of a staffed landline, but I missed physically seeing my daughter and when I tried to call her from the outside courtyard, another patient kept interfering, which curtailed my contact. I was grateful that posters on the ward advertised mental health advocacy and after I reached out to them an advocate attended one of my weekly assessment sessions with the ward psychiatrist and helped me to secure more visitation access to my daughter.*

With very little to occupy them, the service users had to make their own activity, and although some of it was constructive and communal – a game of cards or some sewing for instance – all too often it was destructive, or harmful to themselves and others. Chairs were thrown and broken, whole rooms smashed up, staff attacked or abused. Often the triggers were clear: needing a cigarette, waiting hours to see a nurse or days to see the consultant, frustration at the slow pace of recovery, a cancelled activity. My own principal activity once I had deteriorated so much that I no longer engaged with anything on offer on the ward? Walking up and down endlessly between two points on the walls of my bedroom until my feet began to bleed. Three years and many trips to the chiropodist later, they had recovered so this was a minor offshoot of my illness compared to the deadly activities of some on the ward.

Addressing some of his own mental health issues in a radio interview in 1989, the actor and writer Stephen Fry said that he didn't like the phrase 'cry for help,' which is often used about a suicide attempt. He said that if people need help, they usually shout 'Help!' At the time I thought it was an easy and flippant response to a complex subject. In a way of course, it was, but on that ward in 2020, I saw what he meant. I met people who had long since ceased to cry, let alone ask, for help. They were single-mindedly determined to kill themselves. They discussed it amongst themselves, planned it, prepared for it, waited, did everything they could to dodge the ceaseless observations and then embarked on their deadly plan. First, we hear the alarm, then the dash of nurses along the corridor and into the bedroom. From the door, people watch as CPR is carried out, and a little later the person is helped along the corridor towards the medical room, deep blue/grey marks around their neck. These are things that cannot be unseen, but the people who see them and other horrors day in and day out are the staff, so I want to finish this difficult chapter with them.

The nurses and care assistants who looked after me were exceptionally kind and patient and were all outstanding professionals. They were an eclectic group: young and old: some at the very beginning of this most challenging of careers or getting to the end of a lifetime working on in-patient wards. As Hardcastle (2007) reminds us, 'each member of staff holds their own ideology' (p. 31) and it is important to remember this. *You and your wife just need to talk about decorating the bathroom*, said one senior nurse in a bizarre echo of the 'anti-psychiatry' movement discussed in Chapter 2; *I didn't join the NHS to watch a man the same age as my father behaving like this* said another, younger nurse in a reminder of a harsher approach. It was unkind, but it was the end of a very long day. Like the doctor half a century before telling me I just needed more steel in my spine or the person at the end of the phone saying I just needed more dopamine, these were reminders that in mental health care perhaps above all, the messenger, no matter how highly qualified they are, can only really give a message which is filtered through their own lived experience.

Not all staff on a ward like this of course are nurses, consultants or other clinicians. Far from it. Catering staff, cleaners, volunteers, chaplains, carpenters to repair the doors and windows, social workers, a lot of student nurses and many 'bank' or agency staff. The increasing use of agency staff on NHS mental health wards is a controversial one, but the ones I came across were kind, dedicated and warm. Very occasionally one might doze off briefly on duty, but I knew that some worked poorly paid day shifts in one job and night shifts on the ward in order to support their families.

McCrae and Nolan (2016) found that 'perhaps the most neglected aspect of the history of the mental hospitals is the cultural diversity of the staff' (p. 207). Many on the night shift in my ward were from West Africa. I bonded with a man from The Gambia because my surname is quite common in his country, and apparently I share it with politicians, musicians and famous footballers. We chatted and laughed, and he made me tea. These conversations stay with me as brief moments of warm communion which made me feel good in an otherwise unforgiving environment. Another was with one of the volunteers who had been a patient on the ward in the past and now came back to support the present residents. A courageous act of selfless service to others if ever there was one. We chatted, and it turned out that on Valentine's Day of that year we had both gone to the same pub at the same time with our partners. The food had been inedible, the service poor and all romantic atmosphere lacking. We laughed at this unexpected shared moment of Valentine's Day awfulness from our recent pasts. My mood lifted for the rest of the day.

Sadly, racism was, if not rife, then certainly present: I was sitting next to an older service user and a nurse approached us. This nurse's first name was perfectly matched to his warm and gentle bearing on the ward, and he was admired and loved by his colleagues. He also seemed to work more hours than nearly everyone else and rarely took his statutory breaks. The man next to me abused him with racist epithets now rarely heard. A little later I found myself alone in the corridor with the nurse. *I am so sorry you had to listen to that*, I said. He smiled softly and said:

It's OK. You get used to it.

The staff on that ward put up with a lot: from me, from the other service users but above all from the environment and the system they were working in and continue to work in today. In 2020 of course, they also had to contend with the biggest public health emergency for a century: the Covid-19 pandemic.

Note

1 www.healthwatch.co.uk

References

Fry, S. (1989). Open to Questions. *BBC TV*. May 1st 1989.

Hardcastle, M., Kennard, D., Grandison, S., & Fagin L. (Eds.). (2007). *Experiences of Mental Health In-patient Care Narratives from Service Users, Carers and Professionals*. Hove: Routledge.

Jones, K. (1993). *Asylums and After: A Revised History of the Mental Health Services: From the Early 18th Century to the 1990's*. London: Athlone.

McCrae, N., & Nolan, P. (2016). *The Story of Nursing in British Mental Hospitals: Echoes from the Corridors*. Abingdon: Routledge.

Mumford, J. (2022). Therapy beyond Good and Evil. *The New Atlantis*, 68, 28–38.

6   The impact of the
Covid-19 pandemic

On 31 October 2020, UK Prime Minister Boris Johnson announced a second lockdown to prevent 'a medical and moral disaster for the NHS.' It came into effect on 5 November 2020, and ended partially on 2 December 2020. In Prologue to this book, I mentioned that the five people who took me in that minibus from one provision to another were 'double masked.' This was because that minibus journey took place in December 2020.

This chapter will provide a brief overview of the action taken by some governments and services around the world to mitigate the effects of the pandemic on in-patient mental health settings and a more detailed account of the UK Government's statutory and non-statutory guidance. This will be followed by a discussion of some of the recent research into the impact of the pandemic on in-patient mental health provision. We will also hear two accounts of lived experiences on wards in England in 2020. One of these accounts is the author's own and the other is taken from an extensive interview carried out with Sarah Kingston, a ward manager within an English NHS Trust, who was a charge nurse[1] on an in-patient ward throughout the Covid-19 pandemic.

Duden et al. (2022) conducted a systematic review of 29 early primary studies which reported on mental health services during the Covid-19 pandemic in 63 countries. They found that in Europe amongst heads of psychiatric services, 32% indicated that there had been closures of in-patient units in 2020, with 10.7% acknowledging closures in 2021. In many countries, admission rates decreased during the pandemic. In India, for instance, the number of patients admitted to in-patient services dropped by 76.6% and in Italy by 84.5%. Many in-patient services around the world focused only on emergency cases and some reported early discharges at the beginning of the pandemic for home treatment, though more severely ill patients were generally kept in the in-patient units.

The closure or reduction of in-patient services was related not only to infection control but also to the transformation of former mental health wards to emergency Covid-19 units. Further changes to in-patient services included reducing available beds, as well as restricting patients from leaving the hospital or from receiving visitors. Therapeutic activities within units all round the

DOI: 10.4324/9781003455042-6

world were reduced so that once admitted, patients were less likely to receive treatment. For example, 69.1% of participants indicated a decrease of treatment in Italy and 66% in Brazil.

In England and the devolved nations, several NHS Trusts in the early phase of the pandemic did create dedicated Covid wards within their mental health provision for service users who had contracted the virus. This was very much the experience of Sarah Kingston who described the steps she and her teams took in March and April 2020:

> *We were thinking of course about who could be discharged and at the very beginning we were closed for new admissions, and we did enough discharges to free up one of our two wards as a Covid ward, so up to 16 en-suite bedrooms, though some of these were used for storage of PPE and as changing rooms. The other ward upstairs continued functioning as normal.*
>
> *We created a dedicated Covid team and asked for people to volunteer from amongst the existing staff to be in this team, and it tended to be the younger staff, maybe with no dependents and so not in vulnerable positions.*
>
> *So we made our Covid ward. We had to prepare the ward environmentally at first. At one point, and I'll never have this experience again in my lifetime. I had the strange luxury of about two weeks with an empty ward with no service users on it. So, whilst we were obviously used to responding to alarms and emergency incidents on the ward, this time period of two weeks gave us a chance to practice a new way of responding to alarms: one which involved getting into our PPE (Personal Protective Equipment) really quickly and ensuring that we had apron, gloves, mask and visor. A really strange couple of weeks-productive but very anxiety provoking as we waited. We had the added worry of if the general hospital next door would have enough capacity for its own Covid patients and whether we would have to hand one of our wards over to them.*
>
> *The anxiety of waiting for the first patients on our own Covid ward was quite high because we didn't know what to expect, and if someone came in with Covid we didn't know how ill they were going to be. As mental health nurses we had done aspects of physical nursing but that wasn't really our bread and butter or something we normally have to do every day. We were reading lots of information and trying to learn all sorts of new stuff. Some of the first guidance we received was on CPR (cardiopulmonary resuscitation), which we could all do anyway of course, but that just increased our anxieties.*
>
> *When we did finally have admissions on the Covid ward there was a very different feel to normal, as I was managing only three or four patients so it was actually sort of calmer than before Covid. In the end only a couple of the rooms were used. After a month or so both wards went back to normal.*

From the outset, mental health in-patient wards in the UK followed the Government guidance for general hospitals set out in the document *New Personal*

Protective Equipment (PPE) Guidance for NHS Teams (April 2020) which stipulated that any clinician working in a hospital, primary care or community care setting within 2 metres of a suspected or confirmed Covid-19 patient should wear an apron, gloves, surgical mask and eye protection. In Sarah Kingston's ward, this guidance was only followed in the first months of the pandemic until the need for a dedicated Covid ward had passed:

> At one point in the early days we were in scrubs[2] but not needing to wear masks, but then scrubs went out of the window quite quickly and the use of face masks was in place. We double masked when interacting with patients but not when we were in the office with other staff, but that changed over time too, so we had to double mask in the office as well. It was strange getting used to it to start with but now if anything I find it strange not wearing a mask. We only stopped wearing masks in the last couple of months (June 2023).

Non-statutory guidance covering in-patient wards came from a number of sources, including the NHS itself, the Royal College of Psychiatrists and the British Medical Association, which is the union for many medical workers in the UK, and one senior nurse reflected that at times it was unclear whether guidance had come directly from the Government itself or from the NHS Trust.

In the early weeks of the pandemic, the Oxford Health Biomedical Research Centre, which is part of the Government-funded National Institute of Health Research (NIHR), confirmed:

> Managing infection on a (mental health) ward should mirror the steps taken in the wider community both in trying to prevent spread and the management of any infections. Wards should exercise the principles of social distancing across the ward community. This means minimal contact and an advised distance of two metres. The need to limit contact between individuals should be clearly communicated to patients and staff.

On 27 April 2020, NHS England issued a statement saying that all admissions to all hospitals should be screened using a swab for Covid-19, and those testing positive as well as symptomatic patients should be isolated. Asymptomatic patients awaiting the results of a swab were advised to self-isolate and follow social distancing guidance until results were obtained. On Sarah Kingston's ward, there were times when the nature of a patient's illness made this difficult to manage:

> We had to go through the protocol of using swabs of course. When an individual did test positive, we had to try and manage them and we either looked to manage them in their bedrooms or in different areas of the unit like the 136 suite.[3] There were some service users who did have Covid but

were unable to isolate in their rooms because of their mental health issues, like for instance a lady with bipolar condition who was quite manic at the time and just couldn't retain the information about self-isolating.

NHS advice was that mental health wards that provided single rooms with en-suite facilities should encourage patients to remain in their rooms as much as possible with patients allowed to eat, make phone calls or watch television in their rooms. Staff and patients were encouraged to 'find creative ways to adjust to this' (Oxford Health Biomedical Research Centre, 2020). Activities that normally would bring people into close contact with each other such as ward groups, ward rounds, mealtimes and visiting times were reduced or stopped altogether and although both escorted and unescorted patients leave time off the ward would be maintained as much as possible, it would require additional risk assessment depending on patients' exposure to symptoms while outside the ward. On Sarah Kingston's ward, time slots were allocated for patients to access the courtyard to smoke or simply get some fresh air.

There was a delicate balance to be struck under difficult circumstances between allowing service users on in-patient wards as much autonomy and freedom as possible and the adoption of restrictive interventions to keep people safe. This was particularly challenging with respect to service users detained under the Mental Health Act 1983 during the coronavirus pandemic, so further clarification about this cohort was published online by the NHS in its document *Legal Guidance for Services Supporting People of All Ages during the Coronavirus*, including the following statement:

Health services must continue to have due regard to their obligation to advance equality under the Equality Act 2010, this includes recognising and factoring-in the vulnerability of different cohorts with protected characteristics; and inequalities in access, experience and outcomes in health services (NHS, 2021).

This was certainly the case on Sarah's ward where

the Trust discussed whether it was possible, or ethical, to use the Mental Health Act to force someone to self-isolate if they tested positive for Covid. Most of us felt very uncomfortable with that and in the end the Trust didn't do it.

Emergency changes to the Mental Health Act 1983 legal framework were initially set out in the Coronavirus Act of 25 March 2020 as a last resort should the impact of the pandemic be deemed to be putting patient safety at considerable risk by impeding access to essential care. However, on 30 September 2020, it was announced in Parliament that the Government would seek to remove the Mental Health Act emergency provisions in the

Coronavirus Act. Services were advised to continue to operate in the least restrictive way possible and in accordance with the Mental Health Act and Mental Capacity Act. It was acknowledged that the unprecedented impact of Covid-19 may occasionally result in a justifiable need for restrictive practice in order to maintain both patient and staff safety, such as isolating someone who is suspected or confirmed Covid-19 positive without their consent but that all decisions would be taken on a case-by-case basis, and the provisions of the Equality Act (2010) as set out in the Code of Practice continued to apply to decisions made about patients' care, support and treatment:

- Least restrictive option and maximising independence
- Empowerment and involvement
- Respect and dignity
- Purpose and effectiveness
- Efficiency and equity

In November 2020, the Care Quality Commission (CQC), which is the independent regulator of health and social care in England, in its annual report *Monitoring the Mental Health Act* for 2019–2020 found that 'Mental health services that focused the most on applying the principles of least restriction were more successful in empowering their patients and staff to cope with the extra restrictions imposed during the coronavirus (COVID-19) pandemic' (CQC, 2020).

As early into the pandemic as April 2020, a Royal College of Psychiatrists (RCP) survey found that psychiatrists were being forced to put themselves and their patients at risk, delivering care without adequate PPE or access to tests for themselves, their families or their patients. At one point early in the pandemic, Sarah's ward adopted a *protect the consultants* policy and the consultants conducted their business via video link but in the end this was dropped in favour of safe socially distanced contact in ward rounds. The RCP report found that nearly one in four psychiatrists across the devolved nations didn't have access to correct PPE and that around a quarter (24%) of members were working an 'altered timetable due to reconfiguration of services.' One psychiatrist surveyed said:

There are extreme shortages of PPE and most of us are at risk. Only very limited supply is obtained and most of the time frontline staff are risking their lives. Staff are terrified.

There is already a good deal of academic research into the impact of the pandemic and the successive lockdowns on people's mental health in the community, the impact on children, the impact on people with pre-existing mental health issues and the development of telepsychiatry – or online support – but academic research specifically into the impact on in-patient settings is only just beginning to emerge. We will now though briefly summarise four studies that were undertaken before turning our attention to the lived experience itself.

Benson et al. (2020), writing in *The Lancet Psychiatry* before the development and roll-out of vaccinations, found that 'already there was evidence of rapid spread of Covid-19 in in-patient psychiatric units' (p. 477). They showed that people in mental health in-patient settings were at increased risk of exposure to the virus because of frequent patient and staff turnover and limited space within the wards. They were also at high risk of contracting Covid-19 because their condition may make it difficult for them to recall or in some cases be aware of potential exposures, and 'for a patient presenting with disorganised thinking, determining the date of onset of symptoms may be difficult' (p. 476). Patients in these settings may also 'frequently have underlying medical conditions that worsen their prognosis such as a history of smoking' (p. 476). The article was one of the first to suggest patient separation on the basis of Covid-19 status. On Sarah's ward,

> *we didn't have that many people with Covid, certainly not as many as I had expected, but also because of patient confidentially or because of not wanting to cause an alarm or spread rumours we maybe didn't necessarily tell the other patients if someone had tested positive.*

Writing in the immediate aftermath of the worst of the pandemic, Duden et al. (2022) found that globally, despite many in-patient units restructuring their services to accommodate Covid-19 patients, mental health services had been compromised just at a time when they likely required the most and that this could perhaps have been predicted because research into other major crises, such as the Ebola virus, had shown that these emergencies tended to result in impaired provision of mental health care in particular. They found that 50.5% of professionals in UK in-patient and residential care reported that they could not follow the rules consistently and many experienced limited availability of PPE in mental health services. The study also found that staff experienced changes such as heightened impacts on their own mental health, and a pausing in professional development and training.

Watson and Rowles (2021) looked specifically at the impact on patients detained under the Mental Health Act (1983) who were 'already contending with significant restrictions on their freedom' (p. S300). They conducted structured interviews with 24 service users across the Low Secure and Locked Rehabilitation Division at St Andrews Healthcare in Northampton, England. All participants were detained under the Mental Health Act throughout the pandemic. They found that the patients reported a decline in their mood and that their relationships with loved ones out in the community had suffered from lack of contact, although several participants felt that their relationships with peers had strengthened. Respondents reported that they had had reduced contact with multidisciplinary team members which resulted in delays to their recovery, and that opportunities for escorted time off the ward and exercise had decreased. This has led to an increase in free time and although some used this time to develop hobbies, others reported becoming 'lazy.' The research concluded:

> The pandemic has had significant emotional and psychological effects on society as a whole, but perhaps no group has been more affected than detained patients who have had their lives restricted to a massive degree.
> (p. S300)

A study by Pooja and Driscoll (2020) focused on the potential impacts of the Covid-19 pandemic on in-patient smokers:

> Previously available opportunities to smoke on or near site or when on leave are not available during COVID-19 lockdown, thus disturbing the permissive culture and arrangement between staff and patients of off-site smoking. . . . In mental health hospitals, we are starting to see that the smokefree policies are being relaxed as a quick-fix solution by the health-care practitioners to help their patients cope in the short term and to handle the COVID-19 related challenges.
> (p. 2)

The report recommends smoking cessation 'even during Covid' (p. 1) because 'increased smoking due to Covid-19 threatens to increase the risk of ill health including higher cancer risk in already disadvantaged mental health patients' (p. 2).

In general, then, individual NHS Trusts and wards within those Trusts were largely left to make their own decisions in many areas and to follow statutory and non-statutory guidance as best they could in the very difficult circumstances of the Covid pandemic.

My own experience of the pandemic on the ward described in the previous chapter was very much in line with the findings of the research studies discussed earlier. This was before the widely available test kits which require just a 15-minute wait for the result. The first swab test was carried out on admission after which the patient was isolated in their room for anything between 24 and 72 hours depending on the ability of the lab to return the results. Swabs were carried out every week or so after that, or if there was suspicion of infection, always followed by an isolation period and although I like to think I submitted voluntarily to this isolation, many didn't.

Services were certainly compromised, reduced and impaired but guidance around mask wearing and social distancing could not be followed. In the 12 weeks I spent on one ward, a period which included the second lockdown, I was only aware of one service user who consistently followed all the rules, and it was an impressive achievement. She kept to her own room, only venturing out wearing a mask at the very beginning or end of mealtimes, bringing her own cup and cutlery and carefully positioning herself on her own at a table facing away from everyone else. Caroline, who we heard from in Chapter 5, found the fact that Covid rules were not being followed frustrating at times:

> *We were filling in menus and all sharing a pen. I got really cross because of COVID and demanded that I had a different pen from the office.*

None of the other patients wore masks in any consistent way and most not at all. One older and very distressed man always wore his mask hooked over one ear and dangling down the side of his face. I was not aware of any of the staff ever trying to enforce the rules on mask wearing and this was I think the only possible decision in a place where violence would frequently breakout.

The staff themselves though did mask and usually 'double mask' at all times, but that compromised their ability to maintain any meaningful level of therapeutic communication with the patients. Some staff tried to mitigate the impact of mask wearing on their ability to communicate by fashioning a cheery, laminated photo of their face which they pinned to their chests. A small, but poignant and important gesture. A ward in any hospital though is an airless place and the cleaners, kitchen and maintenance staff in particular suffered enormously in their masks and PPE pushing heavy trolleys around the limited floor space. Everyone has their breaking point though: I had a scheduled 'one on one' with an extraordinarily kind and dedicated nurse. She had worked on this and other wards for years and never flinched from facing a difficult situation. We went into a small side room and sat down at a suitable distance from each other. Well, I sat down. She collapsed into her chair, sat there in silence for a few seconds breathing heavily, then tore off her masks and said:

> *Fuck this, Andrew. I'm sorry. I can't wear these fucking things anymore.*

We carried on, unmasked, but socially distanced.

Rules around social distancing could not apply and were simply not enforced. Visitors were not allowed on the wards at any time, though very occasionally a patient could meet their family in a room away from the ward provided they were socially distanced and supervised. This hit a new young mother on the ward particularly hard. She was unable to see her baby and her self-harm reached terrifying levels.

With the announcement of the second lockdown, the tension on the ward increased noticeably. I was with about 15 other patients and three staff in an art room. We had the radio on and heard the announcement. Most people stopped what they were doing, some became agitated and one dashed out shouting *I've got to get out of here*. I never saw him again. Over the next few days, it was like we were all involved in a sort of sinister lottery as the Multidisciplinary

Teams tried to send the less ill home. Rumours swirled about who was going and who was staying. By then I was so ill I didn't really care. The deadline came and went, and I was still there along with a slightly smaller number of seriously unwell people, supervised by staff, many of them student nurses, but the rooms were soon filled again with new admissions.

The fear of infection was weaponised by a small minority of the more disruptive patients. There were accusations, rumours and demands by patients who were denied leave that those who were able to leave the ward should immediately be isolated for 48 hours on their return. It was also one night during this second lockdown that the ward descended into a violence so extreme that I stayed in bed covered in a sheet because I feared for my life. I am not sure what the trigger was . . . something around smoking probably, but between about 10 p.m. and 2 a.m. there was the constant sound of screams, shouts, windows smashing, doors splintering, alarms sounding, footsteps dashing up and down the corridors. The police arrived but it didn't stop the rioting. I felt certain someone, possibly more than one person, would die.

By early the next morning the ward was quiet again and I ventured outside my room. An extraordinary clean-up had taken place, although there were no chairs left, tables were broken, and wooden panels were being placed over smashed windows and doors. I don't think anyone died that night, but a handful of the more disruptive patients had gone, and never returned.

For some on the ward though, the privations of the pandemic and the restrictions of successive lockdowns went largely unnoticed. Estranged from family and sometimes friendless, the outside world was another country, and many of them didn't want to be in anyway, so with mask wearing and social distancing not enforced, it was simply a case of the usual routines: sleep, eat, medicate, repeat.

Amongst those who felt the full force of that difficult time were the staff: managers, cleaners, care assistants, nurses. Sarah Kingston's professionalism and dedication were clear throughout our interview, but I also asked her to try to give me some idea of her personal experience in the pandemic:

The emotional journey took different forms over the first year. Initially we were really anxious especially as the news at one point seemed to be only about body counts. The greatest anxiety was in the lead up to the first lockdown because we didn't know what to expect, but in the end it was not as bad as we feared and we just sort of got on with it. I had a letter printed out which I would carry in the car with me in case I got pulled over. The letter said you were a key worker for the Trust. So there were times through the pandemic when I actually felt empowered by my role as a key worker in this crisis.

I couldn't see my family, which was strange. I just changed out of my work clothes at the unit, went home, showered and put all my clothes in the laundry, but it feels now like the peak of it didn't last very long.

There were some very difficult moments though. We had a service user who was on one-to-one observations because of the risk to herself. This lady had Covid quite badly actually. She was quite poorly and ended up being admitted to a Covid ward at the General Hospital, which is next door really. But of course, she was still going through her own mental health issues and still on one-to-one observations with us so during that period of time we had to just have a staff group for her over at the general hospital. I remember doing a 7 or 8 hour stint one day, and just sat there next to her because she was a risk to herself if she was left alone. I just had a water bottle but I was on a really intense Covid ward so we had the FFP3⁴ masks and visors, and I could only occasionally take sips of water. The FFP3 masks were really intense and left marks and bruises on your face. Because of supply issues we were told only to use them on our mental health Covid ward for CPR on a patient with Covid due to the amount of air and fluid that procedure would involve. Anyway, by the time I got home I felt really unwell because I hadn't had much to eat or drink and had just been sat in one spot. But it really made me feel for the staff over at the General Hospital who were doing that all the time. That was not a great day.

In May 2022, the British Medical Association undertook a major review into the UK Government's handling of the pandemic and its impact on the NHS as a whole, concluding that the UK Government had failed in its duty of care to protect doctors and the wider healthcare workforce from avoidable harm and suffering in its management of the Covid-19 pandemic.

By the time Prime Minister Boris Johnson announced a third Covid lockdown on 6th January 2021, I was back at home. As I continued to recover in the spring and summer of 2021, I began to reflect on the changes to residential mental health care I had experienced between my first admission in 1985 and my second in 2020, changes which I have tried to summarise and discuss in the preceding chapters. I also experienced the current system under the unique strain of a global pandemic. I was left wondering: what have we gained over the last 40 years in residential psychiatric care, what have we lost, and in fact was it worth closing the asylums at all?

Notes

1 'Charge Nurse' is a term used in both the United Kingdom and the United States to describe a nurse with added responsibilities for supporting a number of other nurses.
2 The word 'scrubs' as used in the United Kingdom and the United States refers to sterile clothing worn by doctors and nurses in clinical settings.
3 A '136 suite' is a facility for people detained under Section 136 of the Mental Health Act (1983) in England and Wales.
4 FFP stands for Filtering Facemask Protection. FFP3 is the highest EU standard for this type of smaller mask and gives a minimum filtration percentage of 99%, and protection against very fine particles.

References

Benson, N. M., Öngür, D., & Hsu, J. (2020). COVID-19 Testing and Patients in Mental Health Facilities. *The Lancet Psychiatry*, 7(6), 476–477.

Care Quality Commission. (2020). *Monitoring the Mental Health Act in 2019–2020: The Mental Health Act in the Covid-19 Pandemic*. London: CQC.

Duden, G., Gersdorf, S., & Stengler, K. (2022). Global Impact of the COVID-19 Pandemic on Mental Health Services: A Systematic Review. *Journal of Psychiatric Research*, 154, (October 2022), 354–377.

NHS. (2021). *Coronavirus " Legal Guidance for Services Supporting People of All Ages during the Coronavirus*. england.nhs.uk (accessed May 21st 2023).

Oxford Health Biomedical Research Centre. (2020). *Inpatient Wards – How to Minimise Risk in Mental Health Inpatient Settings during the COVID-19 Pandemic*. Oxford: NIHR.

Pooja, P., & Driscoll, R. (2020). 'Quit During COVID-19 – Staying Smokefree in Mental Health In-patient Settings. *Ecancer*, 14, ed102. www.ecancer.org; https://doi.org/10.3332/ecancer.2020.ed102

Watson, E., & Rowles, S. (2021). Patient Experiences of the Pandemic; Exploring the Effect of COVID-19 on Patients Detained under the Mental Health Act. *Bjpsych Open*, 7(Suppl 1).

7   From asylums to care in the community

What did we gain and what did we lose?

What has been gained and what has been lost since the closing of the asylums? My own response, based on my experiences in 1985 and 2020, would be cautiously to refer back to Barbara Taylor's warning in 2014, at the end of her book *The Last Asylum*, that it would be 'a tragedy if the death of the asylum means the demise of effective and humane mental health care' (p. 264). Not then, a straight answer, because one person's experience cannot be enough to supply one.

To get closer to a clearer answer, this chapter will draw on recent academic research into in-patient settings, media reporting and official documents, including the Care Quality Commission (CQC) report *Monitoring the Mental Health Act in 2021/22*. The CQC report is based on the findings from monitoring reviews of 609 wards carried out during 2021/22 as well as interviews with 2,667 service users and 726 carers. It also has a dedicated chapter on ward environments.

The chapter will begin with two short accounts of aspects of care in the community today. This book is about in-patient mental health care, but because it was care in the community which replaced the asylums for thousands of former patients, and because care in the community struggled and has been widely criticised almost since its inception, it is important to try at least to get a snapshot of the state of community care today. The term 'care in the community' is of course in reality an umbrella term for a wide range of services, and in this first account I talked to Sarah Weeks, a student nurse enrolled on the MSc Nursing (Mental Health) course at Canterbury Christ Church University in the UK. Sarah also shared with me a paper she wrote in 2023 on Crisis Resolution Home Treatment Teams (CRHT) which she describes as follows:

> CRHT's were formally established in 2000 following the publication of The NHS Plan (2000). The plan called for the introduction of 335 CRHTs to provide a 24-hour, 7 day a week service as an alternative to hospital admission. . . . The crisis team model is comprehensive and fully involves the family and other carers, and the role of the CRHT nurse is to work in partnership with a patient to support them to recognise their existing coping mechanisms.
>
> (Weeks, 2023)

DOI: 10.4324/9781003455042-7

Sarah found that when a patient in crisis is managed in their own home, 'relationships are less dominated by the traditional imbalance of power in healthcare' (ibid.), and so patients not only feel more involved with their care and empowered in their recovery but also learn resilience and other coping skills. However, citing Feldthusen et al. (2022), she finds that staff workloads and shift patterns can impact on a nurse's ability to deliver person-centred crisis resolution in the home, and citing Henderson et al. (2020), she highlights how a professional's anxiety over time pressures, caseloads, lack of resources and risk management can result in care becoming overly outcome orientated. A further significant challenge faced in delivering crisis resolution in the home is staff shortages which can lead to a loss of continuity in the care of the patient. Finally, Sarah makes a point about stigma, a topic which we will address in much more depth the next chapter. She finds that some people 'may be deterred from accepting support from a crisis team due to fears of stigma from neighbours' (ibid.).

The second account of care in the community today is a short case study of 'Alan' (not his real name).

In the late 1970s, Alan spent several months in one of those large and at the time still relatively well-resourced psychiatric hospitals which we discussed in earlier chapters. He was treated successfully, including with electroconvulsive therapy (ECT), and after several months he was discharged and managed his condition for many years, had a career and a family. By the time he suffered a serious relapse about ten years ago, the hospital which had treated him in the 1970s – and may still have treated him today – had long gone. Bulldozed or recycled like all the others.

With no home of his own, Alan is now cared for in the community, which in his case has meant a succession of shared houses, some drab and in poor repair, about 5 miles from the site of the old psychiatric hospital. The back garden of one of these houses was concreted over to save the cost of employing a gardener, and in another Alan was not allowed to access the kitchen to prepare his own meals or even make a cup of tea. His care, and that of others, is managed by two companies with similar names and the same two directors. One company is listed with Companies House as for 'residential letting' and Alan, because he has some savings, pays them a commercial rent. Alan is what is known now as a 'self-funder,' defined by Hudson (2021) as 'individuals who purchase their own support in this new care market' (p. 5). The other company provides healthcare support for Alan and others he lives with under contract to the NHS and they are looked after by staff who provide very little in the way of social or community activities. The healthcare support is inspected by the CQC, but they have no authority to comment on the accommodation as Alan has a private contract with the residential letting company. This is now a common arrangement within care in the community in the UK with private providers again being used to compensate for a lack of public provision.

There are though of course still beds on wards for those whose illness is so severe that they need to be taken into a hospital for more intensive assessment and treatment. However, these beds are becoming more and more scarce. According to the NHS's own statistics, there were 23,515 beds available for people with mental illness at the beginning of the year 2010/2011, compared to 18,029 in the latest period recorded in 2022/2023 (NHS, 2023), which is a decrease of nearly a quarter over 12 years, this despite the fact that the number of people in touch with NHS mental health services has risen consistently over the same period (Campbell, 2021). The CQC report *Monitoring the Mental Health Act in 2021/22*, identifies two of the key impacts of this loss of beds as 'increasing the risk of people ending up in inappropriate environments' (p. 4) and 'placement of people in hospitals out of area' (p. 26), with Campbell (2023) and Savage (2023) both finding that more than 5,000 mental health patients have been sent at least 62 miles from home for treatment and 'a doubling in the number of patients sent more than 300 km (186 miles) from their home' (Campbell, 2023).

This loss of beds has also meant that the NHS in England has had to turn to private providers of in-patient care in a system where 'provision is largely undertaken by private companies' (Campbell & Bawden, 2022). Between 2010 and 2021, while the number of mental health beds in the NHS dropped by more than 5,000, private sector beds paid for by the NHS rose by nearly 1,000:

> The NHS is paying £2bn a year to private hospitals to care for mental health patients which is about 13.5% of the £14.8bn the NHS in England spends on mental health, a dramatic rise since 2005 when it paid £951m. Nine out of every 10 of the 10,123 mental health beds run by private operators are occupied by NHS patients.
>
> (ibid.)

Details of inspections of private providers undertaken by the Care Quality Commission (CQC), and provided to Campbell and Bawden, show that 71 different psychiatric facilities run by non-NHS providers were found to be 'inadequate' since the start of 2017 – more than one in four of the total. We seem to have gone back more than 200 years when, as we saw in Chapter 1, the proliferation of unregulated private 'madhouses' pointed to the need for county asylums funded by the 'poor rates.'

With many less beds in the system as a whole, and much smaller units in NHS facilities, but with no decrease in the incidence of mental illness, mental health care has become the 'fast track system' (p. 251) predicted by Taylor in *The Last Asylum* ten years ago, 'shuttling patients back into the community as quickly as possible' (Jay, 2016, p. 193), a concept often referred to as 'revolving door.' The acute ward, according to Barham (2020), has become essentially 'a warehouse: a relatively safe place where patients can be supervised while the medication kicks in' (p. 2). What this also means, according to Filer (2019), is that 'today people need to be considerably more disturbed before being offered a bed . . . or are discharged much sooner – often before meaningful recovery' (p. 205).

When mental health wards began to be built within or very near to general hospitals some 40 years ago, they were 'designed not unlike the wards of the nearby medical units' (Hardcastle et al., 2007, p. 73): mostly dormitory-type wards intended primarily for short stays. All of the wards I experienced in 2020 had single en-suite rooms, but the 2022 CQC report on ward environments expresses concern over the continued use of dormitories in some settings and 'urge the government to continue to make funding available until all dormitory accommodation has been replaced' (p. 9). The report also expresses general concerns about 'the physical environment and condition of many wards' (p. 1), with their 'plain and institutional feel with bare walls' (p. 3), and in one of its more damning sections comments that 'the very nature of hospital wards, including the lighting, noise levels and general environment, can be non-therapeutic' (p. 7). Barham (2020) goes further:

> So distressing are the ward environments that they may inadvertently provoke violence amongst patients as the only feasible way of attracting attention or communicating.
>
> (Barham, 2020, p. 63)

The problem of chairs being regularly smashed was also not unique to my own experience, with the CQC report finding one ward where 'there were only 6 chairs in the dining area for a ward with 11 beds' (p. 6).

The very limited provision of green space and fresh air is also cited in the CQC report, which describes some of the outdoor spaces visited as 'barren, visually impoverished environments dominated by security fencing' (p. 46). Some patients told them that 'they were regularly unable to get fresh air' (p. 14) with the loss of space and outdoor environments reducing opportunities for exercise. The CQC did though praise one modern facility where patients and relatives commented that the new building is 'such an improvement,' 'amazing,' and 'like a 5-star hotel.' Patients found that 'the service is excellent,' and praised innovations such as touch-screen walls in the seclusion rooms. The provider reported a 60% reduction in violent incidents since the move to the new building.

However, when we compare the fresh air, space and variety of the old asylums with the 'pressure cooker facilities on acute in-patient wards' (Hardcastle et al., 2007, p. 73), the physical environment provided by the old asylums was richer in many ways: there was simply more to do, more to see, more to touch, more to smell, just a more interesting sensory experience. This though of course does not negate one of the defining issues of the old asylums and one which is often cited as being justification enough for their demise: the institutionalisation of those within them.

The man in that ward in Netherne who had stolen a milk bottle 80 years earlier, was certainly 'institutionalised': he and others had nowhere else to go than the institution that was the hospital. But being in an institution is not necessarily the same as being institutionalised, and Jack (1998) found that 'the conventional wisdom that all residential care results in institutionalisation, and that this does not occur elsewhere in the community, is conceptually inadequate' (p. 18). There are plenty of other 'institutions without walls' (ibid., p. 29) and we all live in them at one time or another, but during the three months or so I spent in Netherne Hospital in 1985, it was clear that the hospital had no intention of keeping me any longer than was necessary. I cannot say the same about my time on a ward in 2020. The more time I spent there, the more I felt I might never leave. There were also patients who had been in many times before and who kept coming back: the revolving door phenomenon itself a form of institutionalisation.

Care in the community came to be seen as the cure for institutionalisation (Johnson & Walmsley, 2010) but for many people in the 21st century, 'communities are the stuff of nostalgic dreams' (ibid., p. 111) with 'geographical communities in decline' (ibid., p. 132). The chaotic and isolating home lives of some people with mental illness have been described by Lowe and DeVerteuil (2020) as 'ambiguous home' reflecting the juxtaposition of the home as 'a sanctuary, yet somewhere that is also threatening due to factors such as inability to afford food and heating, poor maintenance and housing insecurity' (Weeks, 2023). In cases such as these, the in-patient ward, for a short period at least, may be the most appropriate place, as it was for a man of about 70 who was in the room opposite to mine in 2020. He could not go home, because he had no appropriate home to go to, but also because he had no clothes, spending the whole day in a pair of paper-thin hospital pyjamas. Eventually, a social worker arrived with a set of second-hand clothes she had got hold of, and he left.

So, to a certain extent at least, the safety and well-being of the man in the pyjamas, though not his dignity, was ensured by an institution and the same could be said for a number of my fellow service users. The ward provided a community of sorts for them. There was a farm worker who as far as I was aware had no visitors and hardly ever spoke, but we did jigsaws together, others joined in, and there was some sense of a community around him. Service user Amy, who we heard from in Chapter 5, had a similar experience:

I think one of the positive aspects of the ward with its regulated mealtimes and expectations was that it offered some patients structure that they desperately needed in their normal lives. I met several regular patients who almost seemed happy to be readmitted, and certainly not shocked by ward norms in the way I was. They had to some extent been institutionalised and treated staff like long-lost friends.

In a study carried out in 2021, Rusca et al. (2022) examined the social networks of people with long-term mental health problems living in the community compared to the in-patient population, and found that

> people with serious and enduring mental health problems living in the community had a significantly greater number of people in their social network than those who were in-patients, but the in-patient group reported greater levels of emotional and practical support from their network.
>
> (p. 1071)

In other words, meaningful socialisation when in hospital is not only possible, but crucial to the well-being of patients: 'relationships are vital to recovery as they shape identity and contribute to well-being' (p. 1071).

Yet, other than jigsaws and occasionally games of cards, that potential for socialisation was barely realised in 2020, and this can only partly be put down to the restriction of successive Covid lockdowns. The CQC report nearly two years after the pandemic laments 'a lack of meaningful activities' (p. 13) on many wards around the country and it is difficult to see any improvement since Hardcastle et al.'s 2007 description of the modern ward experience as not much more than 'excruciating boredom relieved only by mealtimes, medication and the occasional brief 'group' (p. xxiii).

Service user Amy made the point that just because someone needs residential psychiatric help doesn't mean their basic needs can be ignored, but some basic needs do get ignored in the pressure cooker environment of the modern ward. On this, the CQC's findings in 2022 were very much in line with my own and others' experience. They found 'a lack of lockable spaces for people to keep their belongings in' (p. 9) and, possibly more meaningfully for many patients: 'inadequate WiFi access and coverage, limiting people's ability to contact friends, family and advocates' (p. 47).

We must not, of course, ignore the well-being of the staff. We have already seen in Chapter 5 that they are under enormous pressure, subject to violence and abuse, witness terrible things, save lives and have been put under the enormous additional strain of dealing with the Covid-19 pandemic. Where do today's staff go to unwind? Who supports them? Right up to the 1980s, Netherne Hospital in common with other asylums had staff social clubs and sports teams, outings and activities, including a staff drama group. 'The spirit that animated those institutions' (Barham, 2020, p. 3) has disappeared, and has not been replaced. There are also quite simply not enough qualified staff, with the CQC devoting the whole first chapter in its *Monitoring the Mental Health Act in 2021/22* report to 'staff shortages and the impact on patients' (pp. 10–19).

Therapeutic interventions and support on in-patient wards are also getting scarcer, with Noble and Hackett (2023) finding that 'despite recommendations for psychological therapies to be provided on acute inpatient wards there was often limited access to them.' Amy mentioned that she had had one session of art therapy, but that was not in evidence just over a year later, so I asked Maggie Batchelar, a Lead Art Psychotherapist with an English NHS Trust and over 30 years of practice as an Art Therapist, to reflect on what has happened to this provision, which was once at the heart of the therapeutic work of Netherne and other hospitals. She started by underlining the enduring legacy of the work of Edward Adamson more than 40 years ago:

> *The 'enabling space' (Stevens, 1984) provided instinctively by Edward Adamson at Netherne from the 1950s seems to me to be central to contemporary Art Therapy practice in in-patient settings:*
>
>> The consensus in the UK art therapy in-patient literature is that in acute settings the open studio group model offers 'a reliable and constant structure, a flexibility of interaction and withdrawal, as well as a safe emotional place' (Brooker et al., 2007, p. 33). (Marshall-Tierney, 2014, p. 97)
>
> *However, I have seen a lack of commitment to and varying provision for Art Therapy in in-patient settings, despite the National Institute for Care Excellence (2014) recommending Arts Therapies for psychosis and schizophrenia. This is at a cost to many people who are unable at the time of admission to make use of cognitively based 'talking' therapies, due to the disruption in being able to effectively communicate complex, contradictory, distressed states of mind and feeling.*
>
> *The motivation involved in choosing to come to the art therapy space and then of art making are gestures of assertion of self and agency, much of which can become compromised in an inpatient admission. Offering people the space and conditions to*
>
>> make art – and have a close relationship with someone whose role and skill is to see, hear and witness what you say and make – strengthens and draws from the pool of human resilience and capacity to recover.
>> (Learmouth, 2005, p. 18)
>
> *I have though a cautious optimism at the development of thinking around reframing psychological distress away from the narrow, pathologizing diagnostic medical lens to a focus on understanding how our experiences affect and shape us. Art Therapy's values chime with this framework and I am hopeful that this will herald a better understanding of the need for access to all Arts Therapies in in-patient services. I also wonder if mental health services are now beginning to work more attentively with*

people with lived experience who report the need for and benefit from having access to Art Therapy:

> The mental health service user voice has been too long neglected on the basis of 'lack of insight.' The result is a dearth of research into the service user perspective on psychological therapy.
>
> (Woods & Springham, 2011, p. 60)

Despite Maggie's cautious optimism, much has been lost, some historically problematic issues with in-patient mental health care have not gone away, and others have come back. In particular, issues around equality and diversity seem to be persistent and intractable. In 2016, McCrae and Nolan found that concerns had been growing over the 'disproportionate number of black men detained under the Mental Health Act' (2016, p. 223), and according to Filer (2019), 'psychiatry's problematic relationship with Black people stretches back at least as far as slavery in America when a slave might be diagnosed with "drapetomania" – the name given for the mental illness of trying to flee from captivity' (p. 190). Actor David Harewood in his 2021 memoir *Maybe I Don't Belong Here* details through the lens of his own experience the social inequalities linked to race and identity in mental health provision, and the CQC report *Monitoring the Mental Health Act in 2021/22* concludes:

> Despite numerous reports and plans for change, progress in tackling the overrepresentation of people from some ethnic minority groups subject to Mental Health Act powers is too slow.
>
> (p. 8)

We also now seem to have returned to a long-ago age when people we now describe as having learning difficulties are confined to psychiatric wards, with the CQC report finding that 'care for people with a learning disability and for autistic people is still not good enough' (p. 31), and Harris (2023) reporting in *The Guardian* newspaper that the health authorities are 'subjecting hundreds of people to completely the wrong care, and ensuring that many of them are effectively locked up.' It is a situation described with unflinching clarity in Sara Ryan's book, *Justice for Laughing Boy: Connor Sparrowhawk – A Death From Indifference* (Ryan, 2017), about the death of her son, who lived with autism and epilepsy. He drowned aged 19 when he was left unsupervised in a bath on a hospital ward.

Neglect still exists within in-patient settings and has been well documented in places whose names have become synonymous with abuse: The Edenfield Centre, Whorlton Hall, The Deanery Care Home, Winterbourne View Hospital. Writing in *the Guardian* in 2023 about an independent enquiry into the deaths of almost 2,000 mental health patients across NHS trusts, Siddique lists allegations including 'sexual assault against patients, staff taunting or neglect of patients, improper use of restraint, and patients being discharged with insufficient care in place.' Barham (2020) also finds that 'the degradations and indignities associated with mental hospitals were not peculiar to those regimes. They had a nasty habit of reproducing themselves in some of the newly created settings in the community' (p. 48), and referring to the situation in America, Solomon (2014) agrees: 'If major hospitals have been sites of abuse, the chances are that community-based programs will become sites of comparable or worse abuse' (p. 393).

Restraint and restriction are still sanctioned in the UK and many other countries, though with the caveat that care must take place within the least restrictive environment. Butterworth et al. (2022) conducted a systematic review and thematic synthesis using data from 21 qualitative studies of restrictive practices in in-patient wards, with restrictive interventions defined as follows:

> Physical and chemical restraint (e.g. rapid tranquillisation) which aims to restrict movement or control behaviour in an emergency, and seclusion which is intended to isolate and reduce sensory stimulation to calm the patient and ensure everyone is safe . . . a patient's liberty may also be restricted, for example, by disallowing access to outdoor space.
>
> (p. 1)

They found that despite reducing restrictive practices being a priority internationally, restraint and the use of seclusion are widespread with 'patients studied describing persistent post-traumatic-type experiences following a restraint' (p. 4).

Hardcastle et al. (2007) define the history of in-patient care as follows:

> [A] recurring cycle of stages: from neglect to custodial and repressive regimes, on to enlightened and liberal and humane care, and then back to a mixture of neglect and highly regimented and controlled environments.
>
> (p. 8)

We seem now to be in an era and a culture characterised by highly controlled environments where 'risk is the main driver behind day-to-day decision making' (Taylor, 2014, p. 255). Weeks (2023), citing Graney et al. (2020), finds that 'the use of risk assessments provides protection against accusations of poor practice,' but the creation of small highly controlled ward environments with an intense 'emphasis on risk avoidance' (Hardcastle et al., 2007, p. 205) has also led to a curtailment of liberty and choice. In-patient mental health wards are not just for people detained under the Mental health Act: there are still people who enter in-patient provision of their own choice, though usually heavily encouraged by medical professionals. In the UK, these used to be called 'voluntary patients,' though now tend to be called 'informal service users.' The UK-based mental health charity MIND[1] states that one of the key rights of an informal patient is that 'you can leave the hospital when you want, but you are still expected to take part in your treatment plan.' The reality though in my own and others' experience is that free movement to and from the ward environment is so tightly controlled that informal patients cannot easily enact their rights. During my early weeks on the ward in 2020, I thought I would go on regular jogs around the heathland next to the hospital. That would have been my 'choice' – a word which appears 25 times in the NHS *Five Year Forward View for Mental Health* (2016), but first, I had to wait for a nurse to be available to fill in the necessary form, noting exactly what I was wearing, what my state of mind was, exactly where I was going and how I could be contacted. I then had to wait for another nurse to be available to take me through the security doors and along the corridors which led to the outside world. Usually, I just gave up waiting and went back to my room.

Barham (2020) states that 'the void left by the erasure of the old mental hospital regimes has been filled, or compensated for, by a new coercive and fear driven zealotry' (p. 8). 'Zealotry' is a strong word, and not one perhaps I would use, except with respect to one thing. I haven't touched a cigarette since shortly after my discharge from Netherne Hospital in the summer of 1985, but with respect to the blanket ban on smoking in all outside areas in mental health wards, I would describe this unequivocally as zealotry. I have witnessed more violence on the wards triggered by the smoking ban than anything else. People who are in mental health wards don't need punishing further. If a cigarette is one of their ways of coping, that should not be denied them. They can deal with trying to give up when they feel better.

Thirty years ago, Kathleen Jones found that 'nobody really argues for the return of the old mental hospital system; but its abolition has left a chasm between intentions and performance' (Jones, 1993, p. 253). My own and others' experience and an interrogation in this chapter of academic literature, newspaper articles and official reports has shown that this chasm still exists and is arguably wider than before.

Institutions, it turns out, were 'not the only problem, nor did deinstitutionalisation deliver a solution, or possibly the solution was at too high a cost' (Johnson & Walmsley, 2010, p. 82). Care in the community isn't working because it has never been funded properly, but also because, maybe, the community simple doesn't care enough. Writing in 1976, Elizabeth Bott, cited in Barham (2020), suggested that the paradox of the mental hospitals was always that they had been 'in a situation of trying to help an individual on behalf of a society which does not recognise its wish to get rid of the individual as well as to help him' (p. 129) and nearly half a century later, Andrew Solomon was harsher:

> A vacuum of empathy exists in any system that returns people who don't know how to be in the community to communities that may not be prepared to handle them.
>
> (Solomon, 2014, p. 313)

There is though no lack of empathy from the nurses, care assistants, and other staff who daily give of themselves to support patients in the most unforgiving of environments, but, apart from the simple fact that there are not enough beds, many of these wards are simply not conducive to recovery. The community mental health team warned me that the ward I would end up on was *not in a good place right now*, and Barham (2020) agrees that 'the psychiatric wards of the district general hospitals are not the kind of environment which a responsible doctor would want to wish upon anyone' (p. 63), with Muijen (2002) warning that 'it would be surprising if a public service was tolerated when it was feared by its customers' (p. 342).

'The residential mental hospital (Jay, 2016, p. 230), the asylum's last incarnation, has not been done away with. In acute care wards and secure units the locked doors, reinforced glass and the smell of the hospital are still the norm.' When I re-read Kesey's (1962) novel One *Flew over the Cuckoo's Nest*, I was shocked at how many echoes there are in it of my very much not fictional experience in 2020: the staring at blank TV's, the cigarettes as currency, the violence, the bare walls, the tiny plastic mattresses, the waiting for something to do, anything to happen.

Interviewed for BBC Radio 4's 2023 podcast *Is Psychiatry Working?* consultant liaison psychiatrist Chloe Beale, herself a service user, sums up the current system as follows:

> *Excessive coercion based on risk at one end, and exclusion from the system at the other.*

It's a bleak assessment. Something, possibly everything, has to change. In the next chapter, we will look at barriers to that change, and will try to imagine what an effective modern in-patient provision might look like. But I promised to return to what is now 'Netherne Village' and see how the ambitious plans for a sustainable community on the old hospital site turned out.

The developers never built the retirement complex, nursing home, business centre, public house or restaurant and sold much of the land intended for recreational open space to other developers, so the Netherne Village now has over 500 houses and apartments, tastefully converted from the old asylum buildings. In April 2023, the apartment which occupies the top floors of the once infamous water tower sold for a little under half a million pounds. I suspect Enoch Powell would have approved.

The hospital's cemetery remains in a neglected state. The builders could have exhumed the bodies and cleared the site under the Disused Burial Grounds (Amendment) Act 1981 but chose not to on cost grounds. The easiest and cheapest solution was to let it grow wild. The graves of over 1,300 former asylum patients are all but lost in the impenetrable undergrowth. Forgotten in life and forgotten in death.\

Note

1 www.mind.org.uk

References

Barham, P. (2020). *Closing the Asylum – The Mental Patient in Modern Society*. London: Process Press.

Brooker, J., Cullum, M., Gilroy, A., McCombe, B., Mahony, J., Ringrose, K., Russell, D., & Waldman, J. (2007). *The Use of Art Work in Art Psychotherapy with People Who are Prone to Psychotic States: An Evidence-based Clinical Practice Guideline*. London: Oxleas NHS Foundation Trust and Goldsmiths.

Butterworth, H., Wood, L., & Rowe, S. (2022). Patients' and Staff Members' Experiences of Restrictive Practices in Acute Mental Health In-patient Settings: Systematic Review and Thematic Synthesis. *BJPsych Open*, 8, e178; 1–11. https://doi.org/10.1192/bjo.2022.574

Campbell, D. (2021). Number of NHS Mental Health Beds Down by 25% since 2010. *The Guardian*. July 5th 2021.

Campbell, D. (2023). More Than 5,000 Mental Health Patients Sent Over 62 Miles for Treatment. *The Guardian*. June 21st 2023.

Campbell, D., & Bawden, A. (2022). NHS Paying £2bn a Year to Private Hospitals for Mental Health Patients. *The Guardian*. April 24th 2022.

Care Quality Commission (CQC). (2022). *Monitoring the Mental Health Act 2021/22*. https://www.cqc.org.uk/publications/monitoring-mental-health-act

Feldthusen, C., Forsgren, E., Wallström, S., Andersson, V., Löfqvist, N., Sawatzky, R., Öhlén, J. & Ung, E. (2022). Centredness in Health Care: A Systematic Overview of Reviews. *Health Expectations*, 25(3), 885–901. https://doi.org/10.1111/hex.13461

Filer, N. (2019). *This Book Will Change Your Mind about Mental Health*. London: Faber and Faber.

Graney, J., Hunt, I., Quinlivan, L., Rodway, C., Turnbull, P., Gianatsi, M., Appleby, L., & Kapur, N. (2020) Suicide Risk Assessment in UK Mental Health Services: A National Mixed-methods Study. *The Lancet Psychiatry*, 7(12), 1046–1053. https://doi.org/10.1016/s2215-0366(20)30381-3

Hardcastle, M., Kennard, D., Grandison, S., & Fagin L. (Eds.). (2007). *Experiences of Mental Health In-patient Care Narratives from Service Users, Carers and Professionals*. London: Routledge.

Harris, J. (2023). Learning-disabled and Autistic People are being Neglected and Tortured. How Much Longer? *The Guardian*. April 24th 2023.

Henderson, P., Fisher, N., Ball, J., & Sellwood, W. (2020). Mental Health Practitioner Experiences of Engaging with Service Users in Community Mental Health Settings: A Systematic Review and Thematic Synthesis of Qualitative Evidence. *Journal of Psychiatric and Mental Health Nursing*, 27(6), 807–820. https://doi.org/10.1111/jpm.12628

Hudson, B. (2021). *Clients, Consumers or Citizens – The Privatisation of Adult Social Care in England*. Cambridge: Cambridge University Press.

Jack, R. (Ed.). (1998). *Residential Versus Community Care: The Role of Institutions in Welfare Provision*. London: Macmillan Press Ltd.

Jay, M. (2016). *This Way Madness Lies*. London: Thames and Hudson.

Johnson, K., Walmsley, J., with Wolfe, M. (2010). *People with Intellectual Disabilities – Towards a Good Life?* Bristol: The Policy Press.

Jones, K. (1993). *Asylums and After: A Revised History of the Mental Health Services: From the Early 18th Century to the 1990's*. London: Athlone.

Kesey, K. (1962). *One Flew Over the Cuckoo's Nest*. London: Penguin Books.

Learmouth, M. (2005). Changing Our Minds. *Openmind*, 134. July/August 2005.

Lowe, R., and DeVerteuil, G. (2020). The Role of the 'Ambiguous Home' in Service Users' Management of Their Mental Health. *Social & Cultural Geography*, 23(3), 443–459. https://doi.org/10.1080/14649365.2020.1744706

Marshall-Tierney, A. (2014). Making Art with and without Patients in Acute Settings. *International Journal of Art Therapy*, 19(3), 96–106. https://doi.org/10.1080/17454832.2014.913256

McCrae, N., & Nolan, P. (2016). *The Story of Nursing in British Mental Hospitals: Echoes from the Corridors*. Abingdon: Routledge.

MIND. (2022). *Informal Patients. About Informal Patients – Mind* (accessed August 25th 2023).

Muijen, M. (2002). Acute Wards: Problems and Solutions. Acute Hospital Care. *Psychiatric Bulletin*, 26(9), 342–343.

National Institute for Care Excellence. (2014). *Psychosis and Schizophrenia in Adults: Prevention and Management*. Clinical guideline [CG178].

NHS. (2023). *Beds-Timeseries-2010–11-onwards-Q4–2022–23-YQWSA.xls (live.com)* (accessed August 19th 2023).

Noble, J., & Hackett S. (2023). Art Therapy in Acute Inpatient Care. *International Journal of Art Therapy*. https://doi.org/10.1080/17454832.2023.2175003.

Rusca, R., Onwuchekwa, I.F., Kinane, C., & MacInnes, D. (2022). Comparing the Social Networks of Service Users with Long Term Mental Health Needs Living in Community with those in a General Adult In-patient Unit. *International Journal of Social Psychiatry*, 68(5), 1071–1077.

Ryan, S. (2017). *Justice for Laughing Boy: Connor Sparrowhawk – A Death by Indifference*. London: Jessica Kingsley Publishers.

Savage, M. (2023). Mental Health Patients Face Travel Ordeal Despite Minister's Pledge. *The Observer*. May 21st 2023.

Sidique, H. (2023). Essex Mental Health Inquiry Pointless without Legal Powers, Say Families. *The Guardian*. April 7th, 2023.

Solomon, A. (2014). *The Noonday Demon: An Anatomy of Depression*. London: Vintage Books.

Stevens, A. (1984). In Adamson, E. Art as Healing. *Therapy*, 1, 32–36.

Taylor, B. (2014). *The Last Asylum*. London: Penguin.

Weeks, S. (2023). *A Critical Discussion of the Use of Crisis Resolution Home Treatment as an Alternative to In-patient Admission* (Assignment as part completion of an MSc Nursing (Mental Health)). Canterbury: Canterbury Christ Church University.

Woods, A., & Springham, N. (2011). On Learning from being the In-patient. *International Journal of Art Therapy*, 16(2), 60–68.

8 Addressing stigma and building a better future for in-patient mental health care

Mental illness is not going away. We will never eradicate it because 'in reality, the origins of major forms of madness remain almost as mysterious as ever' (Scull, 2015, p. 401). Genetic, environmental, biological, social, domestic factors; unresolved issues in childhood; trauma, poverty, neglect, disease, abuse and much more besides, all acting singly or together on our brain, on our mind, on our emotions. 'The brain is about neurons and neurotransmitters; the mind is about metaphors and meaning' (Hardcastle et al., 2007, p. 194): this much we know – or do we? Do we really know enough, other than that:

> [T]he very shape of the brain, the neural connections that develop and constitute the physical underpinnings of our emotions and cognition are profoundly influenced by social stimulation, by the cultural and the familial environment.
>
> (Scull, 2015, p. 410)

And the environment we live in is not get any easier. Clinical psychologist Sanah Ahsan (2023), writing in *The Guardian* in 2022. put it like this:

> Doesn't it make sense that so many of us are suffering? Of course it does: we are living in a traumatising and uncertain world. The climate is breaking down, we're trying to stay on top of rising living costs, still weighted with grief, contagion and isolation, while revelations about the police murdering women and strip-searching children shatter our faith in those who are supposed to protect us.

Something has to change for the in-patient care of those of us with serious mental illness. It has to change to improve our treatment and recovery, to support the work of the staff and to address the way serious mental illness is perceived. So where do we go from here? What is the answer to that question I didn't answer in the middle of the night after that uncomfortable minibus journey: *How do you think we could improve the service provided to you today?* But first, what are the barriers to meaningful change?

DOI: 10.4324/9781003455042-8

'Secrecy,' Andrew Solomon reminded us in 2012 'is a difficult habit to break' (p. 307). He quotes the novelist Clare Allen:

> There seems to be some sort of agreement, a contract you sign when you first break down, that should you ever emerge from your madness and re-enter the normal world you promise never to mention what took place.
>
> (Solomon, 2012, p. 353)

There is still a 'specific stigma around mental illness' (Hardcastle et al., 2007, p. 69) and we find it very difficult to talk about: I was once employed as a 'poll clerk' in a rural polling station in the UK on the day of an election. There were two of us and we had to stay in that polling station together from 6 in the morning to 11 at night. That was 17 hours in the same room with someone I met for the first time on that day. Voters came in dribs and drabs. Occasionally there was a bit of a rush, but often there were great stretches of time where we were on our own. We got on well, the other polling clerk and me. We chatted easily, shared stories, food, jokes, confidences. We talked about anything and everything, but it was not until the last half hour of those 17 hours together that we somehow found out that we had both at different times been in-patients in the same mental health provision. Why did it take us so long to acknowledge that defining shared experience?

Public attitudes to mental illness remain stubbornly resistant to change and it is can still be the case that 'the reactions around some people with serious mental illness are more distressing than the condition itself' (Filer, 2029, p. 49). There is still a significant mindset that equates mental illness with fault, bad choices, intention, weakness, and this leads, for the person who is or has been ill, to embarrassment, to shame and to silence. Hardcastle (2007) categorises some of the reactions of those around us to our struggles as 'amateur psychoanalysis, desperate pleading and reasoning' (p. 89), and we could add to that trivialisation, anger and blame, such as this comment I once heard: *now you'll be able to see what people who have real problems are like*, as if we have somehow chosen to be like this, to leave our sanity behind, risk losing everything and enter a very terrible tunnel with no visible end.

In 2020, I was lucky. Very lucky. My wife never judged or condemned. She just waited. She said to friends who rang: *I know he'll get better in the end*. Patience and acceptance perhaps all that is required.

Nor are professionals immune from holding stigmatising opinions. Chloe Beale again, consultant liaison psychiatrist and also a service user, speaking on the Radio 4 Podcast *Is Psychiatry working* in 2023:

> *Stigma in the health professions is as much as much of a problem as everywhere else: there's a real hierarchy that has developed in the way health professionals see people with mental health problems or behavioural disturbance. It's either: 'it's behavioural, it's volitional, they know what they*

are doing' and we look down on that, whereas we often view psychosis with more sympathy. We separate the two out and attach a moral judgement to them.

We are more enlightened than that though, aren't we? We talk about mental health more, we have campaigns – we 'open up' – celebrities 'share.' Dobson and Rose (2022) acknowledge that 'the moral imperative to address stigma has been recognized in many countries, and it has also been estimated that stigma reduction and improved use of mental health services are highly cost effective' (p. 27), and yet in a recent study, Schomerus et al. (2022) found that in Germany stigma has become more severe regarding acute schizophrenia, whereas only slightly improving for depression. In contrast, in England, more than ten years of the highly visible *Time to Change* initiative from 2008 to 2021 did bring about an improvement of attitudes towards people with non-specific mental health problems and a growing familiarity with symptoms of depression, but at the same time meant that severe mental illness such as psychotic conditions, or symptoms which cannot be adequately communicated with 'a simple celebrity-headed soundbite' (Filer, 2019, p. 58) look even more unrelatable. Stigma, despite all our efforts, is a complex social process (McKenzie et al., 2022, p. 2) which is proving resistant to treatment.

Central to initiatives to tackle stigma has been 'raising awareness,' including the 'myth and fact' approach in which common myths about mental illness are set against the facts, but in a recent study Dobson and Rose (2022) have shown that this approach may have the reverse effect of re-enforcing the myth. After all, if you suddenly shine a light on something, a lot more people are going to see it.

A number of well-known figures – royalty even – have talked about their mental health in recent years and this can only be a good thing, except, 'openness depends partly on the type of mental health problem being talked about' (Barham, 2020, p. 8). In a 2023 letter to *The Observer* newspaper, consultant psychiatrist Dr Musa Sami writes that despite many campaigns to raise awareness of mental illness, severe conditions such as psychosis, schizophrenia, bipolar disorder, personality disorders, addictions and severe depression still remain a 'neglected group' and this has led to 'systemic discrimination and health inequality.' He concludes: 'Being "aware" of mental health issues is not enough; we need to be mental-health literate so we can prioritise those with the greatest need,' and Filer (2019) agrees: 'campaigns all too often begin and end with raising awareness whilst doing nothing to improve knowledge' (Filer, 2019, p. 56). Perhaps we need to show severe mental illness in all its grimy reality?

Severe mental illness is frequently sordid, dirty, degrading, messy, shameful. You do things which you regret for ever, think apocalyptic thoughts but can't un-think them no matter how hard you try. You suffer in terrible, intangible ways, and people around you suffer. They blame you and they blame themselves. The moment of breakdown, if there is one, is only very occasionally dramatic as often depicted in TV dramas, where the narrative seems to go like this within just one short scene:

> *Blank stare . . . screaming . . . turning over a table or smashing a vase . . . collapsing to the floor and sobbing.*

Severe mental illness is more accurately described by Michelle Thomas in her book *My Sh*t Therapist and Other Mental Health Stories* (2021) like this:

> It's collapsing onto bed, shutting the door on your parents, your loved ones, the people who want to help you, because you're exhausted from carrying the weight of your own worthlessness.

Or by Barbara Taylor in *The Last Asylum* (2014), like this:

> I am starving. Nothing I put inside me satisfies me. I could devour the world, but I chew myself (my nails, my hair) instead. I keep on eating. There is no repletion. Candy bars, vodka, pills: I keep going till I throw up.
> (p. 60)

And if you are a parent, struggling to cope with a child who is ill, you might think this, as quoted by Andrew Solomon in his book *Far from the Tree* (2014)

How do you keep on loving a son who can be an unpleasant stranger?' (p. 329)

Another principal weapon against stigma in recent decades has been to put mental illness on the same footing as physical illness, a concept which as we have seen in earlier chapters, was the rationale behind much of the mass de-institutionalisation of the second half of the 20th century. But is mental illness really the same as physical illness or injury? Many people reject this particular anti-stigma message and Filer (2019) is unequivocal: 'The truth is that mental illness isn't remotely like a broken leg.'

Mental illness should and must be treated with the same rigour and attention, receive at least as much funding as physical injury and illness, but it is not the same as physical injury or illness because when we are mentally ill, that illness effects our whole being: everything we do, everything we think and everything we say. It knows everything we know, as Nathan Filer's protagonist reminds us in his novel *The Shock of the Fall* (2014).

If I break my leg, I tell the person in the ambulance that my leg really hurts. I might even tell them I think it is broken. When we are mentally ill, especially if we are very seriously mentally ill, everything we do, think and say passes through the distorted lenses of that illness. Of course, there are moments of lucidity, moments where we can be objective about our condition, but in the very depths of that illness, these moments are rare. And when we do try to express what we are feeling, the person we are talking to can only listen and respond through the slightly less distorted lenses of their own experience, knowledge and prejudices. The 'steel in the spine' advice, the 'more dopamine' advice. Well intentioned, occasionally helpful, but really just shots in the dark.

Nor is going into an in-patient mental health ward the same as going into a ward in a general hospital. A general hospital is not like home of course, and it's annoying when they wake you up at 6 a.m. to ask you what you want for supper, but at least you are in the right place for now and when most of us go into a general hospital we usually feel we are at the start of a process which we hope will lead to feeling better. This is not the same as entering a mental health in-patient ward.

Mental illness and physical illness are not the same, but they could be more closely aligned, and to do that perhaps we need firstly to address the deficits in public policy.

We have already seen that mental illness is subject to stigma so severe that it has wide-reaching and profound consequences beyond the condition itself, but there is a further level of stigmatisation which perhaps is unique to those who are mentally ill. Barham (2020) calls this: 'the stigmatisation of dependence on the state' (p. 17).

'Laws,' according to O'Shea (2021), 'are important because they determine our perception of people who are mentally ill, their human worth and how they should be treated.' We saw in Chapter 1 that the backdrop to the Mental Health Act of 1983 was the Conservative government's championing of free market economics: privatisation, profit, individualism, less reliance on the state, poverty even as 'the fault of the poor' (Filer, 2019, p. 95). These policies came to be reflected in the wider discourse of society's values, and being a member of that society was determined by agency, choice and the capacity to contribute to what Filer (2019) refers to as the 'neoliberal agenda that began redefining citizens as consumers' (p. 95) and under what Kyoto prize-winning philosopher Martha Nussbaum (2007) calls the 'baneful influence of competition' (p. 39). Government policy across all sectors reflected this: public service provision like health and education became 'consumer-led,' and 'choice became a must-have of 20th century welfare policy' (Taylor, 2014, p. 253). This has influenced the ways in which mental illness has been framed and understood in the UK, and consequently those who appear to lack the capacity for self-determination, those who need higher levels of intervention, those, for instance, who are seriously mentally ill, many of whose fortunes are already 'heavily determined by more pervasive features of the social fabric . . . especially poverty' (Barham, 2020, p. 177), have been largely overlooked in both policy and practice. They remain, along with their carers, on the margins of society. This 'denigrated image of the patient' (Taylor, 2014, p. 146) can only thinly be disguised by a bit of 're-badging' (Hardcastle et al.,

2007, p. 175) as 'client' and 'service user' within something called 'patient-led acre.'

Moving through the mental health system in this country, as we have seen throughout this book, is all too often a demeaning and punitive experience, but it shouldn't be. If you are ill, you are ill. You may be unable to work, you may need to depend on others for a while, forever even, but that should not mean you are a less valued member of society. Taylor (2014) reminds us that adult autonomy is a 'fantasy' (p. 260) anyway, and that people, with or without mental illnesses, depend on other people to live a liveable life (p. 264). We all depend on each other to a greater or lesser degree throughout our lives, and that dependency should be acknowledged, celebrated even, in policy and practice. Filer (2019) interviewed a service user who put it like this:

> People talk about independence . . . no wonder lads in hospital are scared of leaving if they are being told it's all about independence. I don't think it is. Teach them it's about interdependence.
>
> (p. 81)

We have already in previous chapters identified the stagnation of mental health policy in this country over the last 200 years, and in this we are becoming almost unique in Europe. About every three years the World Health Organization (WHO, 2021) updates its *Mental Health Atlas*, which collects and disseminates relevant information about mental health resources across all countries grouped under the six WHO regions: Africa, the Americas, Eastern Mediterranean, Europe, South East Asia and Western Pacific. On page 28 of the 2020 Atlas, there is a table showing the year that stand-alone or integrated policy or plans for mental health provision across these countries were published or last revised. In the Europe region, of 45 countries who reported, only 2% have not updated their key mental health policies since 2007. One of these, of course, is the UK.

Where there have been minor policy amendments, they have almost always been about compulsory detainment, with Barham (2020) concluding that the 1983 Act is essentially flawed because it devotes so much space to compulsory hospital admission and not 'the sorts of capabilities that are needed to deal with problems in a care system in which the community is the primary source of care' (p. 173). It is as if recent education policy, and there have been a lot more Education Acts, commissions and white papers than Mental Health Acts since the end of the Second World War, had been principally about classroom discipline. In fact, it is interesting to note that while the Mental Health Act 1983 barely touches on the nature or practice of mental health care, the Education Act 2011 has sections on the place of education, types of schools, class sizes, the school workforce, qualifications, the curriculum, careers education and much more besides. It seems that policy-makers have asked themselves many times what should go on in a classroom and what values we seek to foster, but not what should go on in a mental health ward. I asked author and Senior Civil Servant John Neil why this might be, and this is what he said:

> *Whilst education has been a political battleground since the 19th century and governments have consistently tinkered with education policy, mental health is entirely different. Education gives us the opportunity to forge the next generation in our likeness, whereas most people make conscious efforts not to think about mental health and there are no votes in improving the treatment of mental illness.*

We have, suggest Warburton and Stahl (2020), 'institutionalised a lack of responsibility, moral judgement, and a lack of compassion' (p. 116), and they hope for 'a modern health delivery system that focusses on prevention, takes responsibility for all patients and has adequate resources when there is a crisis' (p. 117), and by 2022 it seemed like there might just be glimmers of light on the dark horizon.

In 2017, Professor Sir Simon Wessley, regius professor of psychiatry at King's College London, was asked by the then UK Prime Minister Theresa May to lead a new reform of the Mental Health Act for England and Wales. The following year Sir Simon and his team produced their report. Four years later, in June 2022, the Government finally published its Draft Mental Health Act Reform Bill. This draft document was, like the 1983 Act it sought to reform, very much about issues relating to compulsory detention, but within it, were signs of a gentler more holistic in-patient mental health provision.

One of the main drivers of the Draft Bill was to 'prevent people from being detained under section 3 of that Act (admission for treatment) on the basis of autism or learning disability' (p. 2), and there was a section on 'Making Treatment Decisions' which contained commitments not to rely merely on:

(i)   the patient's age or appearance, or
(ii) a condition of the patient's, or an aspect of the patient's behaviour, which might lead others to make unjustified assumptions about what medical treatment might be appropriate for the patient.

(p. 10)

There were sections on 'Appropriate medical treatment: therapeutic benefit' (p. 10), 'A patient's current and future needs' (p. 25), and 'After-care services' (p. 46), and while the word 'well-being' occured only twice and 'recovery' not at all, the word 'care,' with 75 occurrences, appeared more than twice as much as in 1983.

There was then cautious optimism perhaps about the future legislative landscape, but this was just a draft Bill and it still had to be put before

Parliament and then become law, something even Sir Simon Wessley, writing in August 2023 in *The Times* newspaper was concerned about:

> It is now widely believed that this may not happen. Not because of any new problems with the proposals but because the government may have other priorities as we head towards a general election.

Sir Simon was right. On November 7th 2023, King Charles read out in the UK parliament a list of the Acts and Bills to be brought forward in the next year. Despite all the work that had gone over the previous six years, a new or even reformed Mental Health Act was not among them. The wait for meaningful reform goes on.

Generally speaking, the NHS doesn't have to wait years before putting its ideas into practice, and in July 2023 NHS England published *Acute in-patient mental health care for adults and older adults – guidance to support the commissioning and delivery of timely access to high quality therapeutic inpatient care*, which is 'the first time that NHS England has published national policy guidance outlining its vision for inpatient mental health care for adults' (p. 2). It seems to address many of the issues service users have identified in this book as being of concern.

Like the Government's draft but since discarded Bill, it seeks to reduce the number of people with a learning disability and autism in mental health in-patient settings whilst at the same time ensuring 'people are not prevented from accessing or receiving good quality acute mental health inpatient care simply because of a disability, diagnostic label or any other protected characteristic' (p. 2). It also acknowledges that 'people from racialised and ethnic minority backgrounds experience systemic barriers to accessing care and receiving inpatient support that meets their needs' (p. 1) and sets out a number of initiatives to improve services for people from these backgrounds. It also 'seeks to eliminate all inappropriate adult acute mental health out of area placements' (p. 3). It commits to making the mental health ward a 'therapeutic environment which feels feel safe, inviting and accessible by creating "attractive and engaging shared spaces," changing fluorescent lighting for alternatives and 'neutralising smells where possible' (p. 20). It recognises that when people are admitted to hospital, this is often accompanied by feelings of loss of power and control and can be traumatic. It is important that 'services work to ensure that the support that is offered in hospital is underpinned by a trauma-informed approach' (p. 11). In-patient services, it suggests, should offer a full range of multidisciplinary interventions and treatment, including 'care that delivers therapeutic benefit throughout their inpatient stay' and interventions which are meaningful and 'meet the person's holistic needs' (p. 17). It also proposes working 'in a cohesive way with partner organisations to support an effective discharge, so that people are supported to stay well when they leave hospital' (p. 2). There is even a section on 'Staff well-being and psychological safety' (p. 37).

So the NHS at least is trying to make things better for in-patient mental health care, and this will in itself help to reduce the fear and stigma around it. None of this though will happen without proper funding, a topic we haven't addressed in any detail in this book, because it is probably clear by now that there has not been enough money to fund an effective mental health service for many decades, but Faraaz Mohammed, program officer for Mental Health and Rights at the Open Society Foundations, New York, writing in the journal *Health and Human Rights* makes this plea:

> National budgeting for mental health . . . requires a reorientation from a framing of mental health as a purely public health concern to one that recognizes the ways in which well-being is affected by access to livelihoods, freedom from discrimination, belonging in a community, and numerous other factors. This offers the potential to utilize resources more holistically and to make decisions that do not see health as separate from, for example, social protection or education.
>
> (Mohammed, 2020, p. 49)

Faraaz Mohammed also finds that 'the perspectives of people with lived experience of mental health challenges seem to be absent in decision-making' (p. 49). So, I sat down with service user Amy, and we talked about what a truly effective and fully funded in-patient provision might look like.

We started on the outside. Meaningful, safe, attractive outdoor spaces both within and all around a provision are essential to the well-being of patients and staff; they help us feel connected to the outside world, to feel less confined, and yet the settings described in this book had very little open space outside the basic footprint of the building and there was nowhere to go, other than the ward or its bleak courtyard. No gardens, no lawns, no space for growing flowers or vegetables.

Other than the cost of land, the argument for reducing open spaces around a mental health provision may be that it also reduces the risk of patients absconding, but risk factors and risk assessments must be incorporated in the design process for therapeutic spaces such as these, and once the building is occupied, ongoing personalised risk assessments should be used on a case-by-case basis. Assessment of risk should not be used as an excuse for cutting costs.

Moving indoors, those vital first impressions of a ward can all too often make the patient feel like a prisoner, like they are losing their very humanity confronted as they so often are by a succession of locked doors, and then the shock of a bland medicalised environment. When we enter an in-patient ward, we should feel welcomed, not processed, and know that we are entering a place of rest and healing: walls painted, or perhaps even wallpapered, in colours which are bright in some rooms, calming in others; clear signposting and essential notices of course, but mitigated by artwork by patients and staff;

spaces for small and large groups, areas for talking one on one, places for games and TV, with comfortable chairs, and easy access to drinks and snacks. And in your room: a bed big enough for the taller patients and a comfortable mattress. Let us also not forget Ernest White's advice from more than a century ago: *the more glass you have in an asylum, the less you have broken the advice*, so in each room a window large enough to enjoy a view – and a meaningful view as well, not as Amy described *a view of bins and cigarette butts*. This brings us back to smoking: a covered outdoor area where anyone, staff or service users, can smoke. It's an opportunity for talking. Community between staff and patients. Smoking cessation clinics and advice too, for those who want them.

And more, much more, to fill the days: arts therapies of course, easier access to therapists and clinical staff, support for your physical and medical needs, but also music and singing, cooking, games, physical activity, indoor and outdoor sports, massage, dance, social groups. Anything which might make us feel better, even just for a while.

When I began to read the Care Quality Commission's *Monitoring the Mental Health Act 2021/22*, I felt it was a fairly measured and enlightened analysis of some of the issues we have addressed in the book. And then, on page 23, I read this:

> By necessity, seclusion rooms are less welcoming spaces for patients and will rarely meet the standards of other patients' rooms.

I describe my own experience of a seclusion room in the epilogue to this book, so I couldn't disagree with the CQC about seclusion rooms being less welcoming places, but why do they have 'by necessity' to be less welcoming? Earlier in this chapter, we discussed stigma, and a significant mindset that equates mental illness with fault and intention, and how that is a major barrier to improving the service. And yet even the Care Quality Commission, the independent regulator of health and social care in England, buys into that narrative: the more ill you are, the worse you have to be treated. Butterworth et al. (2022), see things differently, and suggest that

> introduction of colour, soft furniture and relaxing music in the seclusion rooms could make seclusion a less unpleasant experience.

People with severe mental illness do terrible things – to themselves – to others – but confinement or seclusion should not make them feel worse either about themselves or about those who have secluded them.

Moving away from the ward environment, improvement in follow-up care after discharge from an in-patient ward must improve because, 'compared with the general population, the risk of death was greater for recently discharged people for each cause of death studied, including suicide, deaths related to drugs and alcohol' (Musgrove et al., 2022, p. 471). Amy's prescription is simple and cost-effective in view of the high price of re-admission:

> *Immediate Intensive follow up with regular one to one contact for as long as it's needed.*

I learnt a lot in those dreadful months at the end of 2020: about myself, but also about the treatment of people with severe mental illness. I have learnt a lot in the writing of this book too, so that perhaps now, finally I have provided answers of sorts to that question that I didn't answer on that bleak December night outside a mental health ward after that minibus journey somewhere in England:

> *How do you think we could improve the service provided to you today?*

References

Ahsan, S. (2023). I'm a Psychologist – and I Believe we've Been Told Devastating Lies about Mental Health. *The Guardian*. September 6th 2022.

Barham, P (2020) *Closing the Asylum – The Mental Patient in Modern Society*. London: Process Press.

Butterworth, H., Wood, L., & Rowe, S. (2022). Patients' and Staff Members' Experiences of Restrictive Practices in Acute Mental Health In-patient Settings: Systematic Review and Thematic Synthesis. *BJPsych Open*, 8, e178, 1–11. https://doi.org/10.1192/bjo.2022.574

Care Quality Commission. (2022). *Monitoring the Mental Health Act 2021/22*. https://www.cqc.org.uk/publications/monitoring-mental-health-act

Dobson, K., & Rose, S. (2022). "Myths and Facts" Campaigns Are at Best Ineffective and May Increase Mental Illness Stigma. *Stigma and Health*, 7(1), 27–34.

Filer, N. (2019). *This Book Will Change Your Mind about Mental Health*. London: Faber and Faber.

Hardcastle, M., Kennard, D., Grandison, S., & Fagin L. (Eds.). (2007). *Experiences of Mental Health In-patient Care Narratives from Service Users, Carers and Professionals*. Hove: Routledge.

McKenzie S., Oliffe J., Black A., & Collings S. (2022). Men's Experiences of Mental Illness Stigma Across the Lifespan: A Scoping Review. *American Journal of Men's Health*, 16(1). https://doi.org/10.1177/15579883221074789

Mohammed, F. (2020). Addressing the Problem of Severe Underinvestment in Mental Health and Well-Being from a Human Rights Perspective. *Health and Human Rights Journal*, 22, 1.

Musa, Dr. S. (2023). Awareness of Mental Health is Not Enough. *The Observer*. May 21st 2023.

Musgrove, R., Carr, M., Kapur, N., Chew-Graham, C., Mughal, F., Ashcroft, D., & Webb, R. (2022). Suicide and Other Causes of Death among Working Age and Older Adults in the Year after Discharge from In-patient Mental Healthcare in England: Matched Cohort Study. *The British Journal of Psychiatry*, 221, 468–475. https://doi.org/10.1192/bjp.2021.176

NHS England. (2023). *Acute Inpatient Mental Health Care for Adults and OLDER ADULTs – Guidance to Support the Commissioning and Delivery of Timely access to High Quality Therapeutic Inpatient Care* (Publication reference: PR00033). London: NHS England.

Nussbaum, M. (2007). *Frontiers of Justice: Disability, Nationality, Species Membership*. Harvard: Harvard University Press.

O'Shea, N. (2021) *Now or Never: A Systematic Investment Review of Mental Health Care in England*. London: Centre for Mental Health.

Schomerus, G., Schindler, S., Sander, C., Baumann, E., & Angermeyer, M. (2022). Changes in Mental Illness Stigma Over 30 Years– Improvement, Persistence, or Deterioration? *European Psychiatry*, 65(1), e78; 1–7. https://doi.org/10.1192/j.eurpsy.2022.2337

Scull, A. (2015). *Madness in Civilization: A Cultural History of Insanity from the Bible to Freud, from the Madhouse to Modern Medicine*. London: Thames and Hudson.

Solomon, A. (2012). *Far from the Tree*. London: Vintage Books.

Solomon, A. (2014). *The Noonday Demon: An Anatomy of Depression*. London: Vintage Books.

Taylor, B. (2014). *The Last Asylum*. London: Penguin.

Thomas, M. (2021) *My Sh*t Therapist and Other Mental Health Stories*. Lerum: Lagom Publishing

Warburton, K., & Stahl, M. (2020). Balancing the Pendulum: Rethinking the Role of Institutionalization in the Treatment of Serious Mental Illness. *CNS Spectrums (2020)*, 25, 115–118. https://doi.org/10.1017/S1092852920000176. Cambridge University Press.

Wessley, S. (2023). It's Finally Time to Reform an Outdated Mental Health Act. *The Times*. August 22nd 2023.

World Health Organization. (2021). *Mental Health Atlas 2020*. Geneva: WHO (Licence: CC BY-NC-SA 3.0 IGO).

Epilogue

Out of the cage

There's not a great deal I can say about the first week or so after I was dropped off in the middle of the night by that minibus at a hospital far from my home. Because I can't remember very much.

I was admitted to a Psychiatric Intensive Care Unit (PICU). Soon after, I was sent to a seclusion room, so I must have done something very bad, but I can't remember what it was. In my defence, I was contacted by a nurse from the same ward months later to thank me for defending her against a very aggressive patient at around the same time, but I don't remember doing that either.

Images from that seclusion room loom large in my nightmares. The Walls: soft and grey. A toilet, and a basin. No bed, just one small thin bare mattress on the floor. That was all. One door with an observation window. Someone sat on the other side of that door and watched me all day and all night. They didn't speak. No other windows, so I had no sense of time. Meals were brought in by two people who put the plate on the floor. No cutlery, so I ate with my hands. The way I had to live in there, I can't bear to think about it. I would beg through the window for tranquilisers, so that I could just go to sleep.

The next stage of my treatment, I have no memory of, so I rely on what I have been told.

I was taken for a round of electroconvulsive therapy (ECT). I have read about ECT since, so I know I would have been told what was going to happen. I may have signed a form giving my consent, or perhaps just my wife signed. I would have been given a general anaesthetic, been strapped to an operating table and then the electric current which was passed through my brain provoked a seizure which, so the theory goes, would begin the process of realigning the electrical impulses in my brain. Except that was not the end of my brain's dramatic activity on that day about a week before Christmas.

During or immediately after the ECT treatment, I suffered a series of transient ischaemic attacks (TIAs), or mini-strokes. I was admitted to the stroke ward of the nearby general hospital. My only memory of those days is a vague visual image of trying to squeeze the fingers of, I assume, a doctor or nurse.

Several days later, when I did start to regain some sort of consciousness of where and who I was, I was back on the PICU, and I realised that, well, I felt a whole lot better. Like seeing that chestnut tree outside my bedroom window in Netherne 35 years before. The relentless catastrophic thoughts, the agitation, the utter despair had gone. After three months of suffering at home, then three months of increasing suffering in hospital, I had, literally come back to my senses.

It soon became clear to the nurses and doctors that I had changed – that I was functioning more or less normally: chatting, noticing, sitting still, listening, even, eventually, laughing. I can't say I enjoyed Christmas Day 2020, but it was certainly better than I had expected it to be. And the food was good.

I was transferred upstairs to a less restrictive ward, and the first thing I noticed was how different it was from the ward described in Chapter 5 of this book. There was no long corridor. The bedrooms were off much shorter corridors which led at different angles from the community areas, which were themselves, well, sort of what you'd expect in a place designed to accommodate for short periods 10 or 15 people who had done nothing wrong: an attractive area for eating, a comfortable area for watching TV or reading, a place for playing table tennis. OK – the outside area was again pretty bleak, and principally used for smoking, but then that was compensated by the fact that there was a kitchen area always staffed by someone, who would make you tea, and give you biscuits and fruit, and chat, whenever you wanted. The nurses' station didn't dominate like it did in the other place. It was there, but kind of faded into the background. Nobody attacked it whilst I was there.

After about a week playing Subbuteo table football with a couple of the other guys on the ward, drinking tea and eating biscuits, the consultant realised that I could probably do all that just as well at home. So, when the time was right, and in the early days of the New Year, I was discharged. I knew again, and still do, that life is worth living.

Index

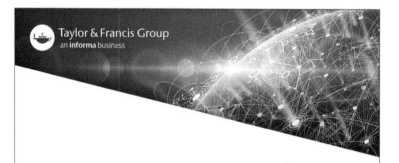

For Product Safety Concerns and Information please contact our EU
representative GPSR@taylorandfrancis.com
Taylor & Francis Verlag GmbH, Kaufingerstraße 24, 80331 München, Germany

www.ingramcontent.com/pod-product-compliance
Ingram Content Group UK Ltd.
Pitfield, Milton Keynes, MK11 3LW, UK
UKHW021055080625
459435UK00003B/12